Health Promotion Theory

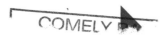

COMELY

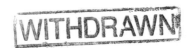

Understanding Public Health

Series editors: Nick Black and Rosalind Raine, London School of Hygiene and Tropical Medicine

Throughout the world, recognition of the importance of public health to sustainable, safe and healthy societies is growing. The achievements of public health in nineteenth-century Europe were for much of the twentieth century overshadowed by advances in personal care, in particular in hospital care. Now, with the dawning of a new century, there is increasing understanding of the inevitable limits of individual health care and of the need to complement such services with effective public health strategies. Major improvements in people's health will come from controlling communicable diseases, eradicating environmental hazards, improving people's diets and enhancing the availability and quality of effective health care. To achieve this, every country needs a cadre of knowledgeable public health practitioners with social, political and organizational skills to lead and bring about changes at international, national and local levels.

This is one of a series of 20 books that provides a foundation for those wishing to join in and contribute to the twenty-first-century regeneration of public health, helping to put the concerns and perspectives of public health at the heart of policy-making and service provision. While each book stands alone, together they provide a comprehensive account of the three main aims of public health: protecting the public from environmental hazards, improving the health of the public and ensuring high quality health services are available to all. Some of the books focus on methods, others on key topics. They have been written by staff at the London School of Hygiene & Tropical Medicine with considerable experience of teaching public health to students from low, middle and high income countries. Much of the material has been developed and tested with postgraduate students both in face-to-face teaching and through distance learning.

The books are designed for self-directed learning. Each chapter has explicit learning objectives, key terms are highlighted and the text contains many activities to enable the reader to test their own understanding of the ideas and material covered. Written in a clear and accessible style, the series will be essential reading for students taking postgraduate courses in public health and will also be of interest to public health practitioners and policy-makers.

Titles in the series

Analytical models for decision making: Colin Sanderson and Reinhold Gruen
Controlling communicable disease: Norman Noah
Economic analysis for management and policy: Stephen Jan, Lilani Kumaranayake,
  Jenny Roberts, Kara Hanson and Kate Archibald
Economic evaluation: Julia Fox-Rushby and John Cairns (eds)
Environmental epidemiology: Paul Wilkinson (ed)
Environment, health and sustainable development: Megan Landon
Environmental health policy: David Ball (ed)
Financial management in health services: Reinhold Gruen and Anne Howarth
Global change and health: Kelley Lee and Jeff Collin (eds)
Health care evaluation: Sarah Smith, Don Sinclair, Rosalind Raine and Barnaby Reeves
Health promotion practice: Wendy Macdowall, Chris Bonell and Maggie Davies (eds)
Health promotion theory: Maggie Davies and Wendy Macdowall (eds)
Introduction to epidemiology: Lucianne Bailey, Katerina Vardulaki, Julia Langham and
  Daniel Chandramohan
Introduction to health economics: David Wonderling, Reinhold Gruen and Nick Black
Issues in public health: Joceline Pomerleau and Martin McKee (eds)
Making health policy: Kent Buse, Nicholas Mays and Gill Walt
Managing health services: Nick Goodwin, Reinhold Gruen and Valerie Iles
Medical anthropology: Robert Pool and Wenzel Geissler
Principles of social research: Judith Green and John Browne (eds)
Understanding health services: Nick Black and Reinhold Gruen

Health Promotion Theory

Edited by Maggie Davies and
Wendy Macdowall

Open University Press

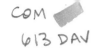

Open University Press
McGraw-Hill Education
McGraw-Hill House
Shoppenhangers Road
Maidenhead
Berkshire
England
SL6 2QL

email: enquiries@openup.co.uk
world wide web: www.openup.co.uk

and Two Penn Plaza, New York, NY 10121-2289, USA

First published 2006

A catalogue record of this book is available from the British Library

ISBN-10: 0335 218407 (pb)
ISBN-13: 978 0335 218370 (pb)

Library of Congress Cataloging-in-Publication Data
CIP data has been applied for

Typeset by RefineCatch Limited, Bungay, Suffolk
Printed in the UK by Bell & Bain Ltd, Glasgow

Contents

Acknowledgements

Open University Press and the London School of Hygiene & Tropical Medicine have made every effort to obtain permission from copyright holders to reproduce material in this book and to acknowledge these sources correctly. Any omissions brought to our attention will be remedied in future editions.

We would like to express our grateful thanks to the following copyright holders for granting permission to reproduce material in this book.

p. 106	Ågren G, *Sweden's new public health policy*. © 2003 Swedish National Institute of Public Health.
p. 117	Arnstein SR, 'Eight rungs on the ladder of citizen participation,' in Cahn SE and Passett BA (eds), *Citizen Participation: Effecting Community Change*, Praeger Publications.
p. 82	Calman KC, 'Cancer: science and society and the communication of risk', *BMJ*, 1996, Vol 313, pp799–802, amended with permission from the BMJ Publishing Group.
p. 166	Chinman M, *Getting to Outcomes 2004*. Copyright RAND.
p. 137	Adapted from Covello V, Message *mapping, risk and crisis communication.* © Vincent Covello 2002.
p. 50	Dahlgren G and Whitehead M, *Policies and strategies to promote social equity in health*, Institute for Futures Studies, 1991. Reprinted by permission of Institute for Future Studies.
pp. 110–11	Henderson P, Summer S and Raj T, *Developing healthier communities. An introductory course for people using community development approaches to improve health and tackle health inequalities*, 2004, Health Development Agency. Reprinted by permission of National Institute for Health and Clinical Excellence.
pp. 161, 163	Kahan B and Goodstadt M, *The IDM Manual: Introduction and basics*, University of Toronto, 2002.
pp. 128, 129	Adapted from Kunreuther H, *The role of insurance in managing extreme events: Implications for terrorism coverage.* Copyright 2002 Howard Kunreuther. Reprinted with permission.
pp. 51–5	*A New Perspective of the Health of Canadians: A Working Document, Health Canada*, 1981 © Reproduced with the permission of the Minister of Public Works and Government Services, Canada, 2005.
pp. 101–2	Markwell S, Watson J, Speller V, Platt S and Younger T, *The Working Partnership – Book 1*, 2003, Health Development Agency. Reprinted by permission of National Institute for Health and Clinical Excellence.
pp. 180–3	Nutbeam D, 'Evaluating health promotion – progress, problems and solutions', *Health Promotion International*, 1998, 13:27–44, by permission of Oxford University Press.

p. 134   Adapted from Sandman P, *Dilemmas in Emergency Communication
                Policy. Emergency Risk Communication CDCynergy (CD-ROM), Center
                for Disease Control and Prevention, U.S. Department of Health and
                Human Services, 2002.

p. 131   Slovic P, Fischoff B and Lichtenstein S, 'Facts and Fears: Understand-
                ing Perceived Risk,' in Schwing R & Albers WA Jr (editors), *Societal
                Risk Assessment: How safe is safe enough?* © 1980 Kluwer Academic/
                Plenum Publishers with kind permission of Springer Science and
                Business Media.

pp. 119–21   Swann C and Morgan A, *Social capital for health: insights from qualita-
                tive research*, 2002, Health Development Agency. Reprinted by
                permission of National Institute for Health and Clinical Excellence.

p. 113   Adapted from Thomas DN, *The making of community work*, 1983.
                Harper Collins.

pp. 21–2   Jakarta Declaration on Leading Health Promotion into the 21st
                century, World Health Organization, 1997. Reprinted with permis-
                sion from the World Health Organization.

pp. 175–7   *Health promotion evaluation: recommendations policy-makers: report of
                the WHO European Working Group on Health Promotion Evaluation.*
                Copenhagen, WHO Regional Office for Europe, 1998. EUR/ICP/IVST
                05 01 03 p. 3–6. http://wwho.dk/document/e60706.pdf

pp. 56, 57–8   Wilkinson R and Marmot M (ed), *Social determinants of health: the
                solid facts 2nd edition.* Copenhagen, WHO Regional Office for Europe,
                2003. pp7–9 and pp: 10, 12, 14, 16, 18, 19, 20, 22, 24, 26, 28.

pp. 170–4   Reproduced with permission from Wimbush E and Watson J, *An
                evaluation framework for health promotion: theory, quality and effective-
                ness.* Copyright (© Sage Publications, 2001), by permission of Sage
                Publications Ltd.

Overview of the book

Introduction

Since the early nineteenth century, the health of the public has improved dramatically, though the extent of such changes has varied between countries and within populations. In high income countries, such improvements have resulted from three main approaches: health care; health promotion, including prevention services; and public policies covering a wide variety of social and environmental conditions. Recently, attempts to quantify the contributions of these different approaches have demonstrated the difficulties of arriving at rigorous conclusions. Despite this, it would appear that the three main approaches have probably contributed equally to the staggering declines in mortality and improvements in people's health that have taken place. This book focuses on the theoretical basis of one of the three main contributors, health promotion.

Focusing as it does on theory, this book is of relevance to low, middle and high income countries. However, given that much of the literature has been produced in high-income countries, there is inevitably an apparent emphasis on those regions of the world. Its important to recognize that most of the ideas and concepts, while originating in high income countries, are equally relevant when considering health promotion initiatives in low and middle income countries.

Why study health promotion theory?

Although it is clear why public health practitioners and students of public health should learn about how to devise and implement health promotion interventions, it may be less obvious why it is necessary to spend time learning about the theory of health promotion. As this book makes clear, health promotion is far from straightforward. Unless public health practitioners explore and understand the theory underpinning health promotion, there is a real risk, at best, of establishing ineffective interventions and, at worst, of antagonizing and even harming the very people you are seeking to help.

This book will guide you through the philosophical, methodological, theoretical, ethical and political underpinnings of health promotion to enable you to be a more effective practitioner. Although the book explores these various aspects, it is firmly focused on assisting you in applying the ideas and concepts to practical implementation of health promotion activities.

Structure of the book

Each chapter follows the same format. A brief overview tells you about the contents, followed by learning objectives and the key terms you will encounter. There are several Activities in each chapter, which are designed to provoke or challenge certain concepts, or to test knowledge and understanding. Each Activity is followed by Feedback to enable you to check on your own understanding. If things are not clear, then you are encouraged to go back and re-read the material. The book consists of four sections, each composed of 3–5 chapters.

Philosophy and theory of health promotion

The book starts by considering such basic questions as: 'What is health?' and 'What is health promotion?' Chapter 1 goes on to consider the historical development of health promotion from its nineteenth-century roots, through health education in the middle decades of the twentieth century, to the emergence of the broader concept encompassed by contemporary health promotion. Chapter 2 brings the story up to date, tracing the key role played by the World Health Organization as well as some important national initiatives, particularly in Canada. You will then turn, in Chapters 3 and 4, to learn about the key theories that have guided health promotion practice at the level of the individual, the community and organizations.

Epidemiology, politics and ethics

Before making use of the theories you have learnt, you need to understand the context in which they are to be applied. The first area of knowledge you need covers the cause and distribution of ill health, the principal aim of epidemiology. In Chapter 5, you will explore the social determinants of health and, in particular, the socio-economic inequalities of health that afflict every country. You will then go on in Chapter 6 to think about the ethical environment in which health promotion inevitably operates, including such thorny issues as the relationship between individuals and the state. The third area that needs thinking about before instituting health promotion programmes is how you are going to know what effect you are having. In Chapter 7, you will consider how to set appropriate targets and standards, the different ways in which targets are set, the data required and the issues that need to be considered, describing the evidence for the impact of targets.

Public policy

Having considered the theoretical basis of your intervention and the environment in which you intend working, you need to consider the policy framework in which the intervention will be introduced. In Chapter 8, building on some of the issues raised in Chapters 1 and 2, you will learn about contemporary concepts of healthy public policy, the constraints it faces and approaches to overcoming them. Then, in Chapter 9, you will see the importance of multi-sectoral and partnership working and the key factors that need to be in place for successful partnerships to be formed. Chapter 10 continues that theme by exploring community development and the concepts of community and social capital.

Implementing health promotion

You are now ready to consider implementing health promotion. Before doing so, you need to consider how your target population is going to perceive your plans. In particular, will they share your perceptions of the risks they currently face? In Chapter 11, you will learn about perceptions of risk and strategies to communicate risk. You will then go on in Chapter 12 to consider the means of motivating behaviour change. This includes the ability to compare and contrast models of health-related behaviour change in terms of the benefits and limitations of the different models. The practicalities of planning a health promotion intervention are considered in Chapter 13, where you will learn about some of the available planning tools.

The task isn't finished yet. You need to know whether your intervention is of any use. In Chapter 14, you will learn why evaluation is important, the particular problems in evaluating health promotion and the different ways impact can be considered. Finally, in Chapter 15, current initiatives to assemble and synthesize what is known about the effectiveness of different health promotion interventions is considered.

Authors

Maggie Davies is Associate Director of Development at the National Institute for Health and Clinical Excellence (NICE); Wendy Macdowall is a Lecturer in Health Promotion, London School of Hygiene & Tropical Medicine; Paul Lincoln is Chief Executive Officer, National Heart Forum; Don Nutbeam is Pro Vice Chancellor, University of Sydney; Antony Morgan is Associate Director of Research, NICE; Nick Fahy is Deputy Head of Unit, European Commission; Jeff French is Director of the National Social Marketing Strategy for Health; Viv Speller is a freelance public health consultant; Magdalene Rosenmöller, Marc Sachon and Jaume Ribera are Professors at the IESE Business School, Barcelona; Mike Kelly is Director of the Centre for Public Health Excellence, NICE; and Jessica Kepford is a freelance consultant.

Acknowledgements

The book is based on the Health Promotion Theory study unit at the London School of Hygiene & Tropical Medicine, which has evolved over several years under the influence of Melvyn Hillsdon, Dalya Marks and many others. The editors are grateful for the comments of Jenny Douglas, Senior Lecturer in Health Promotion at the Open University, and Nick Black, Professor of Health Services Research for editorial input. We also thank Deidre Byrne (series manager) for help and support.

SECTION I

Philosophy and theory of health promotion

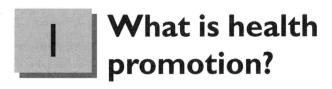

What is health promotion?

Overview

This chapter introduces you to the history and development of health promotion. You will learn about the major influences and movements that have contributed to its evolution from nineteenth-century public health and health education in the middle decades of the twentieth century.

Learning objectives

After working through this chapter, you will be able to:

- **distinguish between public health, health education and health promotion**
- **understand the origins and development of health promotion**

Key terms

Health promotion The process of enabling people to increase control over the determinants of health and thereby improve their health.

Health The state of complete physical, mental and social well-being and not merely the absence of disease or infirmity.

Model Simplified versions of something complex used to analyse and solve problems or make predictions.

Public health The science and art of promoting health, preventing disease and prolonging life through the organized effects of society.

Theory A set of interrelated propositions or arguments that help to clarify complicated problems or help to understand complex reality more easily.

Introduction

Health promotion is probably the most ethical, effective, efficient and sustainable approach to achieving good health. It was defined initially by the World Health Organization in 1986, but the definition has since been refined to take account of new health challenges and a better understanding of the economic, environmental and social determinants of health and disease. The most widely accepted and utilized definition of health promotion is: 'The process of enabling people to increase control over the determinants of health and thereby improve their health' (WHO, 1986).

Before considering where health promotion is located in relation to other public health activities, you first need to think about what is meant by the term 'health'.

 Activity 1.1

Make brief notes on what health means to you.

 Feedback

Health is the most sought after subject on the World Wide Web. The problem of definition is confusing because terms such as health (and education and promotion) are widely used in everyday language and, as such, are used to mean very different things in different contexts. These are essentially contested concepts, as they are used and abused, in the familial sense, in everyday language.

There are two types of definition of health – absolute and relative. The most frequently used absolute definition is that adopted by the World Health Organization in 1946, which defined health as a 'state of complete physical, mental and social well-being and not merely the absence of disease or infirmity'. This may be considered to be idealistic, but it is useful in that it is based on a concept of positive health, not merely the absence of disease. Relative definitions are defined socially and culturally. For example, would most people say that a disabled person could be healthy? Different cultures and societies define states of health very differently – many aspects of health are defined socially and culturally (e.g. neurosis and psychosis). Relative definitions are based on the social and cultural context. Therefore, it is very difficult to define them precisely and thus health is defined in the context in which it is used, rather than in absolute terms.

The emergence of public health

Terms in public health are used differently in different countries and are interpreted differently by politicians, depending upon their ideological perspectives. There is a multitude of terms, including health education, health improvement, health protection, disease prevention and health development. It is important to reflect upon the historical context and the professional and political interests and ideologies that underpin these different concepts. You will explore the origins of these terms and their application by reviewing the history of the development of health promotion.

The term 'health promotion' has a long and complex history. The basis for our current understanding of health promotion can be found in the public health movements of the nineteenth century in Europe and North America. These movements emerged partly in response to a series of major infectious disease epidemics in cities, which had a devastating impact on the population. Improvements in understanding of the mechanisms for the transmission of infectious disease were matched by the actions of social reformers, such as Chadwick and Simon in the UK and Shattuck in the USA, to influence public opinion and promote political action in the form of legislation and regulation to protect the public. These reforms led, in time, to improved housing, sanitation, food supply and working conditions for most of the population.

These advances were secured through political action, often in the face of opposition, and were intended to benefit the entire population, rather than the needs of individuals. Major improvements in the health and longevity of populations in high-income countries were achieved as a consequence of these early public health reforms (McKeown, 1979). This form of societal action has been the cornerstone of public health ever since and is explored in more detail in Chapter 8. It forms the basis for an enduring definition of public health, developed in the 1920s by one of the most influential thinkers and writers on public health, C.E.A. Winslow, who described public health as: 'The science and art of promoting health, preventing disease, and prolonging life through the organized efforts of society' (Winslow, 1923).

Writing in 1923 on the topic of the modern public health campaign, Winslow provided a scholarly analysis of the origins of public health. Of particular significance, he emphasized the beginnings of a new phase in public health where 'education is the keynote of the modern campaign for public health'. He identified the new machinery through which such education could be accomplished as 'health bulletins, health news services, health lecture bureaus and institutes, health cinemas, health exhibits, and health radio programmes'. He further stressed the goals of health education in the context of a public health campaign:

These instruments are all of assistance in their two-fold object, of securing popular support for the community health programme, and for bringing into contact with health clinics various types of individuals who are in need of their services.

Hygienic instruction, plus the organisation of medical services for the detection and the early treatment of incipient disease, these are the twin motives of the modern public health campaign.

Thus, the stage was set for the emergence of health education, together with well-organized preventive health services, as the major tools for the promotion of public health in the middle of the twentieth century.

Post-war development and the expansion of medicine

The lessons learnt in the latter half of the nineteenth century concerning the impact of the physical, social and economic environments became somewhat lost during the two decades following the Second World War. In most high-income countries during this period, a vast amount of investment was made in reconstruction and development. For example, in the UK the National Health Service was created to provide universal access to health care. In the USA, major government initiatives sought to greatly expand the availability of health care facilities and, through the creation of the National Institutes of Health, stimulate a huge expansion in bio-medical research. Further initiatives saw the introduction of Medicare and Medicaid to improve access to health care in the USA for the elderly and the poor.

Through these processes and similar developments in most high-income countries, the role of government in relation to the health of the population became increasingly defined in terms of the availability of and access to health care. The public health perspective was lost. Health education, as it existed in the 1950s and 1960s, remained true to the goals advocated by Winslow, being defined primarily in terms of promoting optimal use of health services, particularly preventive services such as mass screening, ante-natal and child health services, and immunization programmes.

Investment in health care, whether through private health insurance, publicly funded services or a combination of both, grew exponentially throughout the post-war period. Hence, governments in most high-income countries had to develop mechanisms to better regulate the costs of, and to control demands for, health care – a role to which existing skills and programmes in health education could be adapted. A strengthened role emerged for health education, that of encouraging the appropriate use of health services to reduce demand for services. This contrasted strongly with its established role of *promoting* use of preventive health services.

The emergence of health education

Against this background of expansion in medical science and health care, the second half of the twentieth century was characterized by a growth in the importance of chronic, non-communicable diseases as a cause of premature mortality and morbidity, initially in high-income countries and more recently in middle- and low-income countries. Epidemiological studies of this phenomenon have identified individual behaviours or characteristics that are associated with an increased risk of disease. Smoking was the first to receive prominent public attention. Reports from the Royal College of Physicians (1963) in the UK and the Surgeon General in the USA during the 1960s brought this to public attention.

Along with efforts to promote optimal use of health services, modification of such risky behaviour (often referred to as unhealthy lifestyles) increasingly became the focus of efforts to improve public health. Health education was one of the principal tools. So, too, were efforts to encourage people to use preventive health services. The individual and their personal behaviour were the focus for attention, rather than the population and the physical, social and economic environment, the underlying determinants of health that will be considered further in Chapter 5. Since the 1960s, many examples can be found in the literature of health education programmes directed at achieving individual behaviour change. The objectives and target populations varied. These involved, for example, healthy people modifying existing behaviours to reduce present or future risks of disease and injury (for example, by using car seatbelts). In other cases, the target was individuals as patients, directed at promoting optimal use of available health services (for example, by reducing delay in seeking treatment). And in others, it was those who were sick, directed at rehabilitation from illness or the effective management of chronic illness (for example, optimal management of diabetes).

Health education was thus seen not only as offering a solution to the problems of reducing demand for health care but also to a range of emerging threats to individual health. As a strategy health education was seen to be relatively cheap and as health educators mastered the rapidly evolving technologies of mass communication, a relatively high-profile activity – an irresistible combination for politicians.

Development of health education in the 1960s and 1970s

In these circumstances, health education was adopted with enthusiasm and great expectation by governments in countries throughout the world during the 1960s and 1970s. For example, in the UK, a review of health education was conducted between 1960 and 1963. The Cohen Report recommended that a strong central organization be established to:

promote a climate of opinion generally favourable to health education, develop 'blanket' programmes of education on selected priority subjects . . . as well as assist local authorities and other agencies in the conduct of programmes locally. It would foster the training of specialist health educators, promote the training in health education of doctors, nurses, teachers, and dentists and evaluate the results achieved.

(Cohen Committee, 1964)

This report led to the establishment of the Health Education Council in 1968. Establishment of this Council was a major milestone in the evolution of health education in the UK. Together with its successor, the Health Education Authority, it oversaw a large number of health education campaigns (of varying sophistication and success), contributed to the development and training of a specialist group of health education officers throughout the UK, and fostered the development of health education in settings beyond the health system, most notably in schools.

In the USA, in 1973, a President's Committee on Health Education was established to examine opportunities to prevent disease, promote health and improve the capacity of individuals to practise self-care. The report of the Committee examined several options for the organization of initiatives to educate the public on issues concerning health and the appropriate use of health services. Although not clearly linked, this was followed by the establishment, in 1974, of the Bureau of Health Education within the framework of the Centers for Disease Control. This helped develop the scientific basis of health promotion. In 1976, an Office of Health Information and Health Promotion was created within the Federal Department of Human Services and Health, offering a base for the development of health policy. This Office (later renamed the Office for Disease Prevention and Health Promotion), under the outstanding leadership of J. Michael McGinnis, was instrumental in building a firm policy platform for health promotion in the USA.

In several other high-income countries, including Sweden, Finland, Norway, Canada and Australia, health education developed in an *ad hoc* way in the post-war period, closely associated with the evolution of community-based health services. In these countries, health education was organized primarily at local level, often by specialist health educators employed by local authorities and health services. In Australia, for example, such community health services were undeveloped and poorly coordinated until the early 1970s. In 1972, a new Labour government with a mandate for reform promoted the development of community-based integrated primary health care. This was intended to have a strong focus on primary prevention and community participation. Reviews of the community health services in 1976 and 1986 indicate that these services did not develop in the direction, or to the extent, originally envisaged (Baum *et al.*, 1992). However, they provided a strong community-focused base for health programmes and an important counterpoint to a hospital-based, medically dominated health service.

In all the countries mentioned, government interest and investment in health education provided the following: essential infrastructure and resources in terms of a trained workforce; increased capacity to organize both centrally determined and local campaigns; and improved intervention methods achieved through a combination of practical experience and planned research. By the end of the 1970s, many countries had established a central or national governmental agency for health education and some form of local infrastructure for the organization and delivery of community-based health programmes.

The role of non-government organizations

Lest the impression be given that the driving force behind the evolution of health education and health promotion was national governments around the world, it is important to take account of the contributions of non-governmental and community organizations. Many non-governmental health organizations were founded, or developed their activities, during this same period. Organizations such as those concerned with heart disease and cancer raised resources for research and public education and played a leading role in many countries. Typical of these are the Heart Foundations of the USA, Canada and Australia. Philanthropic foundations also contributed significantly. For example, the Rockefeller and Ford Foundations have for many years supported community-based programmes for health, not only in the USA where they are based, but also in many low-income countries. The Kellogg Foundation supported a series of demonstration projects during the 1970s and 1980s. And during the 1980s and 1990s, the Kaiser Family Foundation and Robert Wood-Johnson Foundation made substantial financial commitments to community-based health promotion programmes. Although this form of philanthropic donation is less common in other countries, the contribution of these foundations to the progress of the science and art of health promotion has been immense in the USA.

Reaction and rebellion – self-help and community action

The 1960s and 1970s also saw a rapid expansion in the growth of self-help and self-care groups. These groups were often formed in response to the perception of members that their health care or social support needs were not being adequately met by mainstream health and social services. Generally, they were formed from positions of powerlessness in relation to the health care system which they hoped to overcome (Katz and Bender, 1976). Some groups were part of larger social movements with far wider political aims, such as the women's movement or the civil rights movement in the USA.

Their importance, in relation to the emergence of health promotion, was the desire of such groups to enable individuals to act collectively to exert greater control over their health status and the underlying determinants of health status. The success of these groups was in providing practical and social support for their members, in achieving change and re-orientation in health care provision, and in acting collectively. They provided an important practical example of health promotion in action. Hatch and Kickbusch (1983) reviewed the development and growth of self-help and self-care from a European perspective. Their book captures the essence of this phenomenon, claiming that the growth of interest in self-help and self-care in the 1970s represented a fundamental re-orientation in the system of health care. In particular, they emphasized that self-help is a 'social and not a medical phenomenon' which aims at achieving 'a holistic view of health'. This non-governmental and community-focused dimension to the evolution of health promotion should not be underestimated. In particular, the actions of community organizations have done much to challenge the notion of health promotion as the handmaiden of personal health services. By highlighting the growing dissatisfaction with medically dominated health services, by actively promoting a social view of health and by demonstrating that change could be achieved, the self-help and self-care movements contributed greatly to the development of ideas that were to find their outlet through the Ottawa Charter in 1986, which you will learn about in Chapter 2.

 Activity 1.2

What social and political factors shaped the development of health education and health promotion?

 Feedback

1 The changing nature of the burden of disease – that is, the increase in longevity and the consequential increase in chronic diseases.

2 Increased knowledge about major risk factors for disease, such as tobacco, processed foods high in excess fats, salts and sugars; and the importance of physical activity.

3 Social trends such as the growth in consumerism, self-help and individualism, and 'anti-health' forces such as industries that market health-damaging goods.

4 A realization that the physical, social and political environment shapes people's choices.

5 The changing role and responsibilities of the nation-state, in particular the move from a 'nanny' state to an empowering state, and the development of neo-liberal economic policy.

Health promotion gets a policy platform

A key turning point in the history of what is now referred to as health promotion was the publication in Canada, in 1974, of the Lalonde Report, *A New Perspective on the Health of Canadians*. The report, released by the then Minister for Health, Marc Lalonde, is widely acknowledged as a pioneering statement by a national government. It explicitly recognized that health was created by the complex inter-relationships between biology, environment, lifestyle and the system of health care. Although not greeted with universal praise at the time (Labonte and Penfold, 1981; Labonte, 1994), by giving prominence to the role of lifestyle and the environment in an analysis of public health, the Lalonde Report opened the door to a significant debate in Canada and elsewhere about the role of government in improving health through its policy decisions and the limitations of personal health care. You will look at sections of the Lalonde Report in more detail in Chapter 5 for its emphasis on the determinants of health and again in Chapter 8 for its influence on developing healthy public policy.

Although the Lalonde Report is recognized today for its influence on health policy development, at the time it generated little change in Canada. As Lavada Pinder (1994) succinctly put it, 'there were no announcements, no new resources, and no implementation plan'. It was not until a Health Promotion Directorate was established in the Canadian Federal Department of Health in 1978, under the gifted leadership of Ron Draper, that the ideas put forward in the Lalonde Report began to be considered more systematically.

During this period, the Surgeon General's *Report on Health Promotion and Disease Prevention: Healthy People* (1979) was published in the USA. This provided an overview of the progress in public health in the USA and reviewed contemporary, preventable threats to health. It drew heavily on the growing scientific base of information on health promotion and disease prevention being developed through the National Institutes for Health and identified priority areas in which further gains could be expected over the following decade. In 1985, a mid-term review of progress in the USA showed that the objectives for the nation had helped establish a national health agenda. This was achieved by identifying specific health priorities, facilitating organized responses and supporting progress towards enhanced levels of health. Although the review found that almost half the objectives had been met, it also highlighted the need for further actions to achieve a reduction in some of the major inequalities in health status.

This approach to the development of health policy has continued in the USA. Major review and revision, in 1990, led to the publication of revised goals in *Healthy People 2000*. Such goals and target setting have been adapted as an approach to health policy development by several other countries in the past two decades, including Australia, New Zealand and the UK (Nutbeam and Wise, 1996).

 Activity 1.3

Why did health promotion become a key component of health policy?

 Feedback

The realization that: the escalating cost of health care is unsustainable; the need to reduce demand; the limitation of the power of medicine; and the limited influence of health education. The development of health policy needed to go beyond health care interventions and needed to tackle the causes of ill health and health inequalities.

Summary

You have learnt about the development of modern health promotion from its origins in the nineteenth-century public health measures through the widespread adaptation of health education during and after the Second World War to the emergence of a new paradigm since the 1980s. This has focused on empowerment of people encouraged by statutory services, non-governmental organizations and the self-help movement. However, the principal motivation for the development of health promotion has been the widespread realization of the limited ability of personal health care to solve all the health problems faced by populations.

References

Baum F, Fry D, Lennie I (1992) *Community Health: Policy and Practice in Australia.* Sydney, NSW: Pluto Press

Cohen Committee (1964) *Health Education, Report of a Joint Committee of the Central and Scottish Health Services Councils.* London: HMSO

Hatch S, Kickbusch I (1983) *Self-Help and Health in Europe.* Copenhagen: WHO Regional Office for Europe

Katz AH, Bender E (1976) *The Strength in Us: Self Help Groups in the Modern World.* New York: Franklin Watts

Labonte R (1994) *Death of a Programme, Birth of a Metaphor: The Development of Health.* Place: Publisher

Labonte R, Penfold S (1981) Canadian perspectives on health promotion: a critique, *Health Education* 19(3/4): 4–9

Lalonde M (1974) *A New Perspective on the Health of Canadians.* Ottawa: Ministry of Supply and Services

McKeown T (1979) *The Role of Medicine: Dream, Mirage or Nemesis.* Princeton, NJ: Princeton University Press

Nutbeam D, Wise M (1996) International experiences in health goal and target setting, *Health Promotion International* 11: 219–26

Pinder L (1994) The federal role in health promotion, in Pederson A, O'Neill M, Rootman I (eds.) *Health Promotion in Canada.* Toronto: W.B. Saunders

President's Committee on Health Education (1973) *Report of the President's Committee on Health Education.* New York: Public Affairs Institute

Royal College of Physicians (1963) *Smoking and Health.* London: RCP

US Department of Health and Human Services (1990) *Healthy People 2000: National Health Promotion and Disease Prevention Objectives.* Washington, DC: US Department of Health and Human Services

US Surgeon General (1979) *US Surgeon General's Report on Health Promotion and Disease Prevention: Healthy People.* Washington, DC: US Department of Health and Human Services

Winslow CEA (1923) *The Evolution and Significance of the Modern Public Health Campaign.* New Haven, CT: Yale University Press

World Health Organization, Regional Office for Europe (1986) *Ottawa Charter for Health Promotion.* Geneva: WHO

2 | WHO and international initiatives

Overview

You saw in Chapter 1 how health promotion developed from the nineteenth century up until the 1970s and 1980s. In this chapter, you will learn about the more recent history and, in particular, the key role that the World Health Organization has played through a series of declarations. First, however, you will consider two contemporary models of health promotion that provide a framework for considering such international initiatives.

Learning objectives

After working through this chapter, you will be able to:

- **understand the nature of health promotion in the context of other public health domains and the main democratic political ideologies**
- **understand the need for a multi-sectoral, multi-method and multi-disciplinary approach to health promotion**

Key terms

Primary care Formal care that is the first point of contact for people. It is usually general rather than specialised and provided in the community

Salutogenic Health-producing or -promoting activities.

Introduction: Two models of health promotion

As you have learned in Chapter 1, changes took place in the conceptualization of health and health promotion during the 1980s and 1990s. These have resulted in the creation of several models of health promotion. These will be explored in relation to theory, and to implementation and evaluation of health promotion, in later chapters.

Health promotion is a radical movement, which gathered momentum in the 1980s and which challenges the medicalization of health and stresses the social and economic aspects of health (Downie *et al.*, 1990). Tannahill's model of health promotion sees it as comprising 'efforts to enhance positive health and prevent ill health, through the overlapping spheres of health education, prevention and health pro-

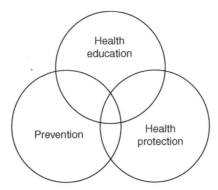

Figure 2.1 Model of health promotion
Source: Downie *et al.* (1990)

tection' (from Downie *et al.*, 1990). Tannahill neatly places health promotion within the framework of the broad range of traditional public health domains. The model can be depicted as a set of overlapping circles with seven domains (Figure 2.1), which are united by the principles of health promotion, the nature of which is eclectic and multidisciplinary. The seven domains are:

- preventive services
- preventive health education
- preventive health protection
- health education for preventive health protection
- positive health education
- positive health protection
- health education aimed at positive health protection

Activity 2.1

1 Review the history of health promotion you learnt about in Chapter 1 from the point of view of the seven domains of the model.
2 Can you track which elements were dominant in different phases of health promotion's history?
3 Considering the health system of your country, which domains are dominant now and where is health promotion practice situated?

Feedback

You should have been able to track the rise and fall of different phases of health promotion over the years using this model and noting the way in which health promotion increases its breadth with the increasing recognition of the multifactorial influences on health. You may also have noted that, in your own situation, different domains have dominance and may be led by different professional groups within public health. In many countries, there is a professional separation in the practice of health protection and health promotion, although both are considered to be aspects of public health.

There are three basic approaches (models) to improving health based on medical/ behavioural change, educational change or social change. In practice, these models overlap but can be described separately to show their differences. First, the medical model focuses on the prevention of disease (illness or negative health) and is combined with a philosophy of compliance with professionals' (usually the doctor's) diagnosis and prognosis. Second, the educational model is based on the view that the world consists of rational human beings and that to prevent disease and improve health you merely have to inform or educate people about remedies and healthy lifestyles because, as rational human beings, they will respond accordingly. And third, the social model is based on the view that health is determined by the social, cultural and physical environment. In this model, solutions are political and require protecting people from health-disabling environments. Like all models, these are simplifications of reality and as such are all incomplete. In practice, health promotion is a combination of these approaches.

The role of the World Health Organization

Health for All (1978)

While the World Health Organization (WHO) has fostered and supported health education and disease prevention programmes around the world throughout its fifty-year history, these efforts were largely uncoordinated and lacked a strategic reference point until the *Health for All* strategy adopted by WHO in 1978 declared:

> The main social target of governments, international organisations and the world community in the coming decades should be the attainment by all peoples of the world by the year 2000 of a level of health that will permit them to lead a socially and economically productive life.

This prompted a significant re-orientation of the work of WHO and, for the first time, provided a comprehensive and coherent strategy for the organization and member states (WHO, 1981). *Health for All* has been important in making equity and social justice major social goals. It has also been credited with fostering a resurgence of interest in public health internationally, particularly by re-focusing attention on social and economic determinants of health and their unequal impact on the health of populations.

Primary health care (1978)

The adoption of the *Health for All* strategy by WHO was followed by what has become recognized as a landmark meeting, jointly organized by the WHO and UNICEF, at Alma Ata, in Kazakhstan. This meeting resulted in the *Declaration of Alma Ata* on primary health care (WHO, 1978), which, like the *Ottawa Charter* that followed, has proved to be an inspirational statement, highlighting the need to reorient health systems in many countries towards the provision of primary health care. Primary health care was defined as: 'Essential health care based on practical, scientifically sound and socially acceptable methods and technology made universally accessible to individuals and families'. The Declaration emphasized that such essential health care:

includes, at least education concerning prevailing health problems and the methods of preventing them and controlling them . . . involves all related sectors . . . demands the co-ordinated efforts of all those sectors . . . and requires and promotes maximum community and individual self reliance and participation in the planning, organisation, operation and control of primary health care.

This focus on primary health care, prevention, recognition of the role of other sectors in creating health and causing ill health, and of community participation and ownership of health programmes has been important to the work of WHO. It has been particularly influential in the evolution of health systems in many low-income countries but, disappointingly, national health policies that reflect the aspirations of *Health for All* and the *Declaration of Alma Ata* have been slow to materialize in high- and middle-income countries with established, medically oriented health care systems.

Targets for Health for All 2000 (1986)

The European Region of WHO has sought to interpret the *Health for All* concept into one more meaningful for the countries of Europe. WHO has promoted a common approach to health policy in Europe by developing a series of targets for improved health status that reflect the *Health for All* strategy – *Targets for Health for All 2000* (WHO, 1986a). This report provided a clear statement of the scope for improving health status within member countries and called for a fundamental reorientation of the health systems in individual countries towards the achieve-ment of the targets. The report grouped targets into four major themes:

- lifestyles and health
- risk factors affecting health and the environment
- reorientation of the health care system
- the infrastructure support necessary to bring about the desired changes in these three areas.

The document recognized the importance of structural prerequisites for health by setting targets for resource allocation, public policy and workforce training. The report also emphasized the need to engage and reorient health systems towards the provision of appropriate care, in particular stressing primary health care as the basis for the health system.

Altogether, 38 targets were specified, together with 65 'essential' regional indicators (or groups of indicators) that could be used to measure progress. Progress reports in relation to the targets are submitted to the WHO every three years by the individual member states and the existence of the targets and reporting mechanisms has meant that these issues are regularly exposed in a public forum.

Ottawa Charter (1986)

Parallel with these developments, the European Office of WHO also sponsored a series of meetings to explore the concept and principles of health promotion, culminating in the organization of the Ottawa Conference on Health Promotion in Developed Countries. The *Ottawa Charter*, which emanated from this meeting, has defined health promotion action in many countries since this time (WHO, 1986b).

Since 1986, WHO has played a leading role in health promotion throughout the world, both by sponsoring international conferences to explore practical experience of the major strategies of the *Ottawa Charter* and by promoting a 'settings'-based model for health promotion. Two WHO conferences that have extended our knowledge and understanding of the strategies defined in the *Ottawa Charter* were held in Adelaide, Australia to examine international experience in developing healthy public policy (WHO, 1988), and in Sundsvall, Sweden to explore ways and means of creating supportive environments for health (WHO, 1991). In the latter case, WHO has supported the development of the Healthy Cities Project, a network of health-promoting schools, and action to support the development of health-promoting worksites and health-promoting hospitals.

The *Ottawa Charter* define health promotion as 'The process of enabling people to increase control over the determinants of health and thereby improve their health'. This salutogenic view implies strengthening people's health potential and that good health is a means to a productive and enjoyable life. Human rights are fundamental to health promotion and a concern for equity, empowerment and engagement. In addition, it has the following characteristics:

- health promotion is a process – a means to an end
- health promotion is enabling – done by, with and for people, not imposed upon them
- health promotion is directed towards improving control over the determinants of health

The *Ottawa Charter* identified a set of five mechanisms:

- building healthy public policy
- creating a supportive environment
- strengthening community action
- developing personal skills
- reorientating health services

These were updated in the *Jakarta Declaration* (WHO, 1997), which focused on creating partnerships between sectors, including private–public partnerships (you will learn more about these methods of multi-sectoral working in Chapter 9). The priorities for the twenty-first century were to:

- promote social responsibility for health
- increase investment in health development
- consolidate and expand partnerships for health
- increase community capacity and empower the individual
- secure an infrastructure for health promotion

More recently WHO, through the Bangkok Charter (2005) has reviewed the strategies for health promotion in a globalised world as the context for health promotion has changed markedly since the Ottawa Charter. In particular, increasing health inequalities, environmental degradation, new patterns of consumption and communication, and increasing urbanisation.

Activity 2.2

The following extract from the Jakarta Declaration considers the influential themes of *Health for All* and the *Ottawa Charter.*

1 Having read it, what needs to happen where you are?
2 How might the perspectives from high, middle and low income countries differ?

Priorities for health promotion in the 21st century

1. Promote social responsibility for health

Decision-makers must be firmly committed to social responsibility. Both the public and private sectors should promote health by pursuing policies and practices that: avoid harming the health of individuals; protect the environment and ensure sustainable use of resources; restrict production of and trade in inherently harmful goods and substances such as tobacco and armaments, as well as discourage unhealthy marketing practices; safeguard both the citizen in the marketplace and the individual in the workplace; include equity-focused health impact assessments as an integral part of policy development.

2. Increase investment for health development

In many countries, current investment in health is inadequate and often ineffective. Increasing investment for health development requires a truly multi-sectoral approach including, for example, additional resources for education and housing as well as for the health sector. Greater investment for health and reorientation of existing investments, both within and among countries, has the potential to achieve significant advances in human development, health and quality of life. Investments for health should reflect the needs of particular groups such as women, children, older people, and indigenous, poor and marginalized populations.

3. Consolidate and expand partnerships for health

Health promotion requires partnerships for health and social development between the different sectors at all levels of governance and society. Existing partnerships need to be strengthened and the potential for new partnerships must be explored. Partnerships offer mutual benefit for health through the sharing of expertise, skills and resources. Each partnership must be transparent and accountable and be based on agreed ethical principles, mutual understanding and respect. WHO guidelines should be adhered to.

4. Increase community capacity and empower the individual

Health promotion is carried out by and with people, not on or to people. It improves both the ability of individuals to take action, and the capacity of groups, organizations or communities to influence the determinants of health. Improving the capacity of communities for health promotion requires practical education, leadership training, and access to resources. Empowering individuals demands more consistent, reliable access to the decision-making process and the skills and knowledge essential to effect change. Both traditional communication and the new information media support this process. Social, cultural and spiritual resources need to be harnessed in innovative ways.

5.   Secure an infrastructure for health promotion

To secure an infrastructure for health promotion, new mechanisms for funding it locally, nationally and globally must be found. Incentives should be developed to influence the actions of governments, nongovernmental organizations, educational institutions and the private sector to make sure that resource mobilization for health promotion is maximized. 'Settings for health' represent the organizational base of the infrastructure required for health promotion. New health challenges mean that new and diverse networks need to be created to achieve inter-sectoral collaboration. Such networks should provide mutual assistance within and among countries and facilitate exchange of information on which strategies have proved effective and in which settings.

Training in and practice of local leadership skills should be encouraged in order to support health promotion activities. Documentation of experiences in health promotion through research and project reporting should be enhanced to improve planning, implementation and evaluation. All countries should develop the appropriate political, legal, educational, social and economic environments required to support health promotion.

Call for action

The participants in this Conference are committed to sharing the key messages of the Jakarta Declaration with their governments, institutions and communities, putting the actions proposed into practice, and reporting back to the Fifth International Conference on Health Promotion.

In order to speed progress towards global health promotion, the participants endorse the formation of a global health promotion alliance. The goal of this alliance is to advance the priorities for action in health promotion set out in this Declaration. Priorities for the alliance include: raising awareness of the changing determinants of health; supporting the development of collaboration and networks for health development; mobilizing resources for health promotion; accumulating knowledge on best practice; enabling shared learning; promoting solidarity in action; fostering transparency and public accountability in health promotion.

National governments are called on to take the initiative in fostering and sponsoring networks for health promotion both within and among their countries. The participants call on WHO to take the lead in building such a global health promotion alliance and enabling its Member States to implement the outcomes of the Conference. A key part of this role is for WHO to engage governments, non-governmental organizations, development banks, organizations of the United Nations system, interregional bodies, bilateral agencies, the labour movement and cooperatives, as well as the private sector, in advancing the priorities for action in health promotion.

Feedback

1 Clearly, your priorities will depend on the state of development and the health problems in your country. The likelihood is that you would want action to take place in each of the five areas identified. However, limited resources (not just financial, but political, human and other) would preclude you pursuing all the actions you would favour, so you would have to decide on priorities.

2 The perspectives from high-, middle- and low-income countries will differ from the different health problems they face. For example, there is considerable investment in health development in high-income countries, not only in health care but also in health protection and preventive services, so the priority might be to promote greater social responsibility for health, particularly within the private industrial sector. In contrast, in low-income countries, additional resources might be the top priority.

Summary

You have seen how the World Health Organization has developed the concept of health promotion since the 1970s through a series of international meetings and declarations. These have helped provide support to individuals and organizations in nation-states to develop health promotion.

References

Downie RS, Fyfe C, Tannahill A (1990) *Health Promotion Models and Values*. Oxford: Oxford Medical Publications

World Health Organization (1978) *Primary Health Care: Report of the International Conference on Primary Health Care*. Geneva: WHO

World Health Organization (1981) *Global Strategy for Health for All by the Year 2000*. Geneva: WHO

World Health Organization (1986a) *Targets for Health for All 2000*. Copenhagen: WHO Regional Office for Europe

World Health Organization (1986b) *Ottawa Charter for Health Promotion*. Geneva: WHO

World Health Organization (1988) *Adelaide Statement on Healthy Public Policy*. Geneva: WHO

World Health Organization (1991) *Sundsvall Statement on Creating Supportive Environments for Health*. Geneva: WHO

World Health Organization (1997) *The Jakarta Declaration on Leading Health Promotion into the 21st Century*. Geneva: WHO

World Health Organization (2005). Bangkok Charter for Health Promotion in a Globalized World. Geneva: WHO

3 Using theory to guide changing individual behaviour

Overview

In this chapter you will gain an overview of the use of theory to guide decision making in health promotion, drawing upon several of the most influential theories and models that have guided health promotion practice in the recent past and which remain influential. You will see how, when used prudently, theories can greatly enhance the effectiveness and sustainability of health promotion programmes.

Learning objectives

After working through this chapter, you will be able to:

- identify ways in which the use of theory can help you understand the nature of the health problem being addressed
- describe and explain the needs and motivations of the target population
- explain or make propositions concerning how to change health status, health-related behaviours and their determinants
- inform the methods and measures used to monitor and evaluate a health promotion intervention

Key terms

Behaviour Actions, activities or conduct of people.

Health belief model One of the first models of health behaviour change which focuses on the individual's calculation of risks and benefits.

Motivation Incentives or driving forces that encourage the adoption of health-promoting behaviours or lifestyles.

Socio-economic determinants Social and economic factors that influence health.

Introduction

Not all forms of public health intervention are equally successful in achieving their aims and objectives. Experience tells us that health promotion programmes are most likely to be successful when the determinants of a health problem or issue are well understood, where the needs and motivations of the target population are addressed, and the context in which the programme is being implemented has been taken into account. That is, the programme 'fits' the problem.

Although many health promotion projects and programmes are developed and implemented without overt reference to theory, there is substantial evidence from published research demonstrating that the use of theory will significantly improve the chances of success in achieving pre-determined programme objectives (Green and Kreuter, 1999; Nutbeam and Harris, 2004).

Theory

As you saw in Chapter 1, theory can be defined as systematically organized knowledge applicable in a relatively wide variety of circumstances devised to analyse, predict or otherwise explain the nature or behaviour of a specified set of phenomena that could be used as the basis for action (Van Ryn and Heany, 1992). A fully developed theory would explain:

- The major factors that influence the phenomena of interest, for example those factors that explain why some people are regularly active and others are not
- The relationship between these factors, for example the relationship between knowledge, beliefs, social norms and behaviours such as physical activity
- The conditions under which these relationships do or do not occur. How, when and why relationships exist, for example, the time, place and circumstances which, predictably, lead to a person being active or inactive.

Using theory in practice

Most health promotion theories come from the behavioural and social sciences. They borrow from disciplines such as psychology and sociology and from activities such as management, consumer behaviour and marketing. Such diversity reflects the fact that health promotion practice is not only concerned with the behaviour of individuals but also with the ways in which society is organized and the policies and organizational structures that underpin social organization.

Many of the theories commonly used in health promotion are not highly developed in the way suggested in the definition above, nor have they been rigorously tested when compared, for example, with theory in the physical sciences. For these reasons, many of the theories referred to below are more accurately termed 'models'.

The potential of theory to guide the development of health promotion interventions is substantial. There are several different planning models that are used by health promotion practitioners. Internationally, the best known of these planning models is the PRECEDE/PROCEED model developed by Green and Kreuter (1999).

Several variations of this approach have also been produced (Nutbeam, 2001). This and other planning models are described in more detail in Chapter 13. In each case, these models and guidelines follow a structured sequence including planning, implementation and evaluation. Reference to different theories can guide and inform practitioners at each of these stages. Figure 3.1 provides a summary of the linkages between the five distinct phases in the process, namely:

- problem definition
- solution generation
- capacity building
- health promotion actions
- outcome measurement

The use of theory in each of these stages is considered in turn.

Problem definition

Identification of the parameters of the health problem to be addressed may involve drawing on a wide range of epidemiological and demographic information, as well as information from the behavioural and social sciences and knowledge of community needs and priorities. Here, different theories can help you identify *what* should be the focus for an intervention.

Specifically, theory can inform your choice for the focus for the intervention. This might be individual characteristics, beliefs and values that are associated with different health behaviours and that may be amenable to change. (Models of behaviour change will be explored in more detail in Chapter 12.) Alternatively, the focus might be organizational characteristics that may need to be changed.

Solution generation

The second step involves the analysis of potential solutions, leading to the development of a programme plan which specifies the objectives and strategies to be employed, as well as the sequence of activity. Theory is at its most useful here in providing guidance on how and when change might be achieved in the target population, organization or policy. It may also generate ideas which might not otherwise have occurred to you.

Different theories can help you understand the methods you could use as the focus of your interventions; specifically by improving understanding of the processes by which changes occur in the target variables (i.e. people, organizations and policies), and by clarifying the means of achieving change in these target variables. For example, *theory* may help explain the influence of different external environments and their impact on individual behaviour. These insights will help in the design of a programme, for example by indicating how changes to the environment can have an impact on health behaviour.

Thus, those theories that explain and predict individual and group health behaviour and organizational practice, as well as those that identify *methods for changing* these determinants of health behaviour and organizational practice, are worthy of close consideration in this phase of planning. Some theories also inform decisions on the *timing and sequencing* of your interventions in order to achieve maximum effects.

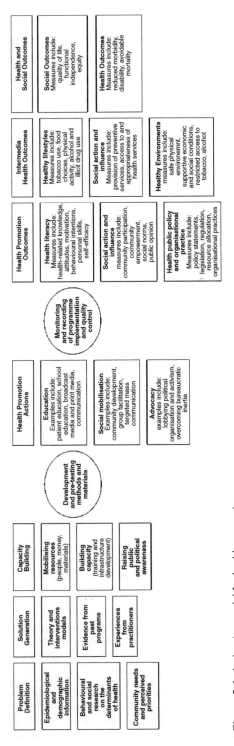

Figure 3.1 A planning model for health promotion

Source: Nutbeam (2001)

Capacity building

Once a programme plan has been developed, the first phase in implementation is usually directed towards generating public and political interest in the programme, mobilizing resources for programme implementation, and building capacity in organizations through which the programme may operate (e.g. schools, worksites, local government). Models theories which indicate how to influence organizational policy and procedures are particularly useful here, as too is *theory* which guides the development of media activities.

Health promotion actions

The implementation of a programme may involve multiple strategies, such as education and advocacy. Here, the key elements of theory can provide a benchmark against which *actual* selection of methods and sequencing of an intervention can be considered in relation to the *theoretically* ideal implementation of programmes.

In this way, the use of theory helps you to understand success or failure in different programmes, particularly by highlighting the possible impact of differences between what was planned and what actually happened in the implementation of the programme. It can also assist in identifying the key elements of a programme that can form the basis for disseminating successful programmes.

Outcomes

Health promotion interventions can be expected to have an impact initially on processes or activities such as participation and organizational practices. Theory can provide guidance on the appropriate measures that can be used to assess such activities. For example, where theory suggests that the target of interventions is to achieve change in knowledge or changes in social norms measurement of these changes becomes the first point of evaluation. Such impact measures are often referred to as *health promotion outcomes* (note, not outcomes in the sense of improvements in health – see below).

Intermediate outcome assessment is the next level of evaluation. Theory can also be used to predict the *intermediate health outcomes* that are sought from an intervention. Usually these are modifications of people's behaviour or changes in social, economic and environmental conditions that determine health or influence behaviour. Theories can predict that health promotion outcomes will lead to such intermediate health outcomes.

Health and social outcomes refer to the final outcomes of an intervention in terms of changes in physical or mental health status, in quality of life, or in improved equity in health within populations. Definition of final outcomes will be based on theoretically predicted relationships between changes in intermediate health outcomes and final health outcomes.

Table 3.1 summarizes the areas of change and the theories or models underpinning them to support the planning, execution and evaluation of health promotion programmes. This chapter introduces you to some important theories used to guide individual behaviour change. Others will be introduced in later chapters.

Table 3.1 Areas of change and the theories or models underpinning them

Areas of change	Theories or models
Theories that explain health behaviour and health behaviour change by focusing on the individual	• Health belief model • Theory of reasoned action • Transtheoretical (stages of change) model • Social learning theory

Theories that explain change in communities and community action for health	• Community mobilization
	  – Social planning
	  – Social action
	  – Community development
	• Diffusion of innovation

Theories that guide the use of communication strategies for change to promote health	• Communication for behaviour change • Social marketing
Models that explain changes in organizations and the creation of health-supportive organizational practices	• Theories of organizational change • Models of intersectoral action
Models that explain the development and implementation of healthy public policy	• Ecological framework for policy development • Determinants of policy making • Indicators of health promotion policy

Source: Nutbeam and Harris (2004)

Selecting an appropriate theory

Theories are not static pronouncements that can be applied to all issues in all circumstances. In health promotion, some of the theories that have been used have been extensively refined and developed in the light of experience. The range and focus of theories has also expanded over the past two decades from a focus on the modification of individual behaviour, to recognition of the need to influence and change a broad range of social, economic and environmental factors that influence health alongside individual behavioural choices.

Thus, health promotion operates at several different levels:

• individual
• community
• organization
• nation

Choosing the right approach is moderated by the nature of the problem, its determinants and the opportunities for action. Programmes that operate at multiple levels, such as those described in the *Ottawa Charter for Health Promotion* (WHO, 1986), are more likely to address the full range of determinants of health problems in populations and, thereby, have the greatest effect.

Activity 3.1

Consider a programme to improve the uptake of a childhood immunization. Suggest some interventions that could be implemented at the level of the individual, the community, the organization of services, and at the national level.

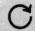
Feedback

- Education to inform and motivate individual parents to immunize their children
- Facilitation of community debate to change perceptions concerning the safety and convenience of immunization
- Changes to organizational practice to improve notification systems and provide more conveniently located clinics
- Financial incentives for parents and doctors

It follows that no single theory dominates health promotion practice and nor could it given the range of health problems and their determinants, the diversity of populations and settings, and differences in available resources, skills and opportunity for action among practitioners.

Depending on the level of an intervention (individual, group, organization or nation), the type of change (simple, one-off behaviour, complex behaviour, organizational or policy change), different theories will have greater relevance and provide a better fit with the problem. None of the theories or models presented in this book can simply be adopted as the answer to all problems. Most often, you benefit by drawing upon more than one of the theories to match the multiple levels of the programme being contemplated.

To be useful and relevant, the different models and theories have to be readily understood and capable of application in a wide variety of real-life conditions. Although you are constantly reminded that 'there is nothing so practical as a good theory', you may remain somewhat suspicious of the capacity of intervention theories to provide the guidance necessary to develop an effective intervention in a complex environment.

Glanz *et al.* (2002) offer a commonsense summary of how to judge a good fit between a theory (or combinations of theories) and the problem you are trying to address. Is it:

- logical?
- consistent with everyday observations?
- similar to those used in successful programmes?
- supported by past research?

Theories and models are simplified representations of reality – they can never include or explain all of the complexities of individual, social or organizational behaviour. However, while the use of theory alone does not guarantee effective programmes, the use of theory in the planning, execution and evaluation of programmes will enhance the chances of success. One of the greatest challenges for you is to identify how best to achieve a fit between the issues of interest and established theories or models which could improve the effectiveness of a programme or intervention.

Three widely used models

One of the major roots of health promotion can be found in the application of health psychology to health behaviour change. Evidence for this can be seen in the phenomenal growth in the discipline of health psychology and the evolution of the concept of behavioural medicine. This discipline has had a significant influence. For several decades researchers have sought to explain, predict and change health behaviour by the development and application of theories and models evolving from psychology and, in particular, social psychology. Among the many theories and models that have been proposed, you will learn about three in the rest of this chapter.

The health belief model

This is one of the longest established theoretical models designed to explain health behaviour by understanding people's beliefs about health. It was originally articulated to explain why individuals participate in health screening and immunization programmes, and has been developed for application to other types of health behaviour.

At its core, the model suggests that the likelihood of an individual taking action for a given health problem is based on the interaction between four types of belief (Figure 3.2). The model predicts that individuals will take action to protect or promote health if:

- they perceive themselves to be susceptible to a condition or problem
- they believe it will have potentially serious consequences
- they believe a course of action is available which will reduce their susceptibility, or minimize the consequences
- they believe that the benefits of taking action will outweigh the costs or barriers.

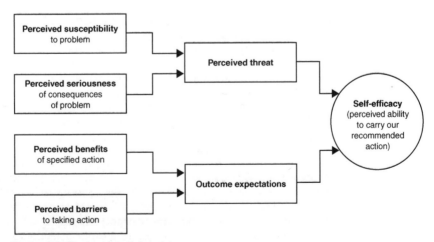

Figure 3.2 The health belief model

Source: Nutbeam and Harris (2002)

Activity 3.2

> If this model was used to shape a public education programme for HIV prevention, what beliefs would it be necessary for people to adopt so as to minimize their risk of infection?

Feedback

> Individuals would need to:
>
> - believe that they are at risk of HIV infection
> - believe that the consequences of infection are serious
> - receive supportive cues for action which may trigger a response (such as targeted media publicity)
> - believe that risk minimization practices (such as safe sex or abstinence) will greatly reduce the risk of infection
> - believe that the benefits of action to reduce risk will outweigh potential costs and barriers, such as reduced enjoyment and negative reactions of their partner
> - believe in their ability to take effective action, such as following and maintaining safe sex behaviours

Studies have shown how the use of a postcard to remind parents of immunizations that are due for their children are effective in raising immunization rates. Hawe and colleagues (1998) examined any difference in impact on immunization rates of using the health belief model to guide the content of a simple postcard message to encourage parents to bring their children for immunization with that of a standard card that provided only the time and place of the immunization clinic. This simple modification, guided by the health belief model, produced a significant improvement in the uptake of immunization in the community in which it was tested.

The health belief model has been found to be most useful when applied to behaviours for which it was originally developed, particularly prevention strategies such as screening and immunization. It has been less useful in guiding interventions to address more long-term, complex and socially determined behaviours, such as alcohol and tobacco consumption. The model's advantage is the relatively simple way in which it illustrates the importance of individual beliefs about health and the relative costs and benefits of actions to protect or improve health. Three decades of research have indicated that promoting change in beliefs can lead to changes in health behaviour which contribute to improved health status. Changes in knowledge and beliefs will almost always form part of a health promotion programme and the health belief model provides a reference point in the development of messages to improve knowledge and change beliefs, especially messages designed for use by the mass media.

The stages of change (transtheoretical) model

This model was developed to describe and explain the different stages in behaviour change (Prochaska and DiClemente, 1984). The model is based on the premise that

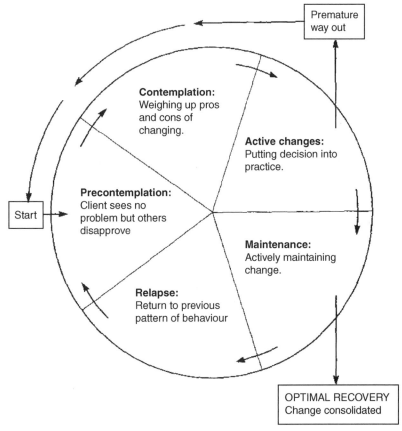

Figure 3.3 The stages of change (transtheoretical) model

Source: Prochaska and DiClemente (1984)

behaviour change is a process, not an event, and that individuals have different levels of motivation or readiness to change (Figure 3.3). Five stages of change have been identified:

- *Precontemplation:* this describes individuals who are not even considering changing behaviour or are consciously intending not to change
- *Contemplation:* the stage at which a person considers making a change to a specific behaviour
- *Determination,* or preparation: the stage at which a person makes a serious commitment to change
- *Action:* the stage at which behaviour change is initiated
- *Maintenance:* sustaining the change, and achievement of predictable health gains. *Relapse* may also be the fifth stage

From a programme planning perspective, the model is particularly useful in indicating how different *processes of change* can influence how activities are staged. Several processes have been consistently useful in supporting movement between stages. These processes are more or less applicable at different stages of change. For example, awareness raising may be most useful among *pre-contemplators* who may not be aware of the threat to health that their behaviour poses, whereas communication of the benefits of change and illustration of the success of others in changing may be important for those contemplating change. Once change has been initiated at the action stage, social support and stimulus control (for example, by avoiding certain situations or having environmental supports in place) are more important.

By matching stages of behavioural change with specific processes, the model specifies how interventions could be organized for different populations, with different needs and in different circumstances. The stages of change model stresses the need to research the characteristics of the target population, the importance of not assuming that all people are at the same stage, and the need to organize interventions sequentially to address the different stages that will be encountered.

The model has been used in workplace programmes to promote regular physical activity, which traditionally have met with limited success. Marcus and colleagues (1992) tested an intervention that used the stages of change model to classify workers according to their current level of activity and motivation to change. The intervention consisted of a mix of written materials and events that were targeted according to the different stage of change. The intervention produced promising short-term results by supporting many participants to move on through the different stages of change towards more regular activity.

 Activity 3.3

Identify three different forms of intervention that would assist individuals to move from their current stage in physical activity to the next stage.

 Feedback

There are several forms of intervention you may have suggested. For example, the provision of gym facilities might assist a person moving from 'contemplation' to 'determination' – that is, a commitment to take action.

The stages of change model has quickly become an important reference point in health promotion interventions because of its obvious advantage in focusing on the change process. The model is important in emphasizing the *range of needs* for an intervention in any given population, the *changing needs* of different populations, and the need for the *sequencing* of interventions to match different stages of change. It illustrates the importance of tailoring programmes to the real needs and circumstances of individuals, rather than assuming an intervention will be equally applicable to all.

Social cognitive theory

This is one of the most widely applied theories in health promotion because it addresses both the underlying determinants of health behaviour and the methods of promoting change. The theory was built on an understanding of the interaction that occurs between an individual and their environment (Bandura 1995). Early psycho-social research tended to focus on the way in which an environment shapes behaviour, by making it more or less rewarding to behave in particular ways. For example, if at work there is no regulation on where people are able to smoke cigarettes, it is easy to be a smoker. If regulations are in place, it is more difficult and, as a consequence, most smokers smoke less and find such an environment more supportive for quitting.

Social cognitive theory indicates that the relationship between people and their environment is more subtle and complex. For example, in circumstances where a significant number of people are non-smokers and are assertive about their desire to restrict smoking in a given environment, even without formal regulation, it becomes far less rewarding for the individual who smokes. They are then likely to modify their behaviour. In this case, the non-smokers have influenced the smoker's perception of the environment through social influence.

This is referred to as *reciprocal determinism*. It describes the way in which an individual, their environment and behaviour continuously interact and influence each other. An understanding of this interaction and the way in which (in the example) modification of social norms can impact on behaviour offers an important insight into how behaviour can be modified through health promotion interventions. For example, seeking to modify social norms regarding smoking is considered to be one of the most powerful ways of promoting cessation among adults.

Added to this basic understanding of the relationship between the individual and the environment, a range of personal cognitive factors form a third part to this relationship, affecting and being affected by specific behaviours and environments. Of these cognitions, three are particularly important. First, the capacity to learn by observing both the behaviour of others and the rewards received for different patterns of behaviour (*observational learning*). For example, some young women may observe behaviour (such as smoking) by people whom they regard as sophisticated and attractive (*role models*). If they observe and value the rewards that they associate with smoking, such as sexual attractiveness or a desirable self-image, then they are more likely to smoke themselves – their *expectancies* in relation to smoking are positive. Such an understanding further reinforces the importance of taking account of peer influences and social norms on health behaviour, and of the potential use of role models in influencing social norms.

Second, the capacity to anticipate and place value on the outcome of different behaviour patterns (referred to as *expectations*). For example, if you believe that smoking will help you lose weight and you place great value on losing weight, then you are more likely to take up or to continue smoking. This understanding emphasizes the importance of understanding personal beliefs and motivations underlying different behaviour, and the need to emphasize short-term and tangible benefits. For example, young people have been shown to respond far more to the short-term adverse effects of smoking (bad breath, smelly clothes) than to any long-term threat posed to health by lung cancer or heart disease.

Finally, the theory emphasizes the importance of belief in your own ability to successfully perform a behaviour (referred to as *self-efficacy*). Self-efficacy is proposed as the most important prerequisite for behaviour change and will affect how much effort is put into a task and the outcome of that task. The promotion of self-efficacy is thus an important task in the achievement of behaviour change. It has been proposed that both *observational learning* and *participatory learning* (e.g. by supervised practice and repetition) will lead to the development of the knowledge and skills necessary for behaviour change (*behavioural capability*). These are seen as powerful tools in building self-confidence and self-efficacy.

Summary

You have learnt about theories that explain health behaviour and health behaviour change. Theories that focus on the individual provide important guidance on major elements of health promotion programmes. Taken together, the theories and models described emphasize the importance of knowledge and beliefs about health, the importance of self-efficacy (the belief in one's competency to take action), the importance of perceived social norms and social influences related to the value an individual places on social approval or acceptance by different social groups, and the importance of recognizing that individuals in a population may be at different stages of change at any one time. There are limitations to psycho-social theories which do not adequately take account of socio-economic and environmental conditions and it is therefore important to change the environment or people's perception of the environment if health promotion is to be successful.

References

Bandura A (1995). Self-efficacy in changing societies. New York: Cambridge University Press

Glanz K, Lewis FM, Rimer BK (2002) *Health Behaviour and Health Education: Theory, Research and Practice*. San Francisco, CA: Jossey-Bass

Green LW, Kreuter MW (1999) *Health Promotion Planning: An Educational and Environmental Approach*. Mountain View, CA: Mayfield

Hawe P, McKenzie N, Scurry R (1998) Randomised controlled trial of the use of a modified postal reminder card on the uptake of measles vaccination, *Archives of Disease in Childhood* 79: 136–40

Marcus BH, Rossi JS, Selby VC, Niaura RS, Abrams DB (1992). The stages and processes of exercise adoption and maintenance in a worksite sample. Health Psychology 11: 386–95

Marcus BH, Banspach SW, Lefebvre RC, Rossi JS, Carleton RA, Abrams DB (1992). Using the stage of change model to increase the adoption of physical activity among community participants. American Journal of Health Promotion 6:424–9

Nutbeam D (2001) Effective health promotion programmes, in Pencheon D, Guest C, Meltzer D, Muir Gray JA (eds.) *Oxford Handbook of Public Health Practice*. Oxford: Oxford University Press

Nutbeam D, Harris E (2004) *Theory in a Nutshell: A Practical Guide to Health Promotion Theories*. Sydney, NSW: McGraw-Hill

Prochaska JO, DiClemente CC (1984) *The Transtheoretical Approach: Crossing Traditional Boundaries of Therapy*. Homewood, IL: Dow Jones Irwin

Van Ryn M, Heany CA (1992) What's the use of theory?, *Health Education Quarterly*, 19(3): 315–30

World Health Organization (1986) *Ottawa Charter for Health Promotion*. Geneva: WHO

4 Using theory to guide changing communities and organizations

Overview

Many of the factors that influence health and health-related behaviour can be traced to social structures and the social environment – the local community in which people live. For these reasons, understanding these social structures, and how to engage and mobilize local communities, is important in health promotion.

Learning objectives

After working through this chapter, you will be able to:

- **explain the relevance of social structures to health-related behaviour**
- **explain the importance of engaging and mobilizing local communities in health promotion practice**

Key terms

Community A society, the population of a specific area, or groups of people. Can also refer to a neighbourhood, district or any centre of population.

Organizational capacity The human resources and management systems that an organization has.

Organizational climate The personality of an organization; those characteristics that distinguish one organization from another, based on the collective perceptions of those who live and work in it.

Organizational culture A set of values and assumptions about an organization.

Social environment The settings, surroundings or atmosphere in which social groups or individuals live, work and interact.

Social structures Ways in which society is organized, configured and constituted.

Introduction

Previously, the community was often seen simply as a collection of individuals, or a means through which it was possible to reach large numbers of people to bring about large-scale health behaviour changes, an easier approach than individual forms of intervention. Many early community programmes, such as the Stanford Heart Programmes in the 1970s, could be characterized in this way. However, communities are now viewed as dynamic systems with inherent strengths and capabilities that can be influenced and supported in ways that will improve health (Nutbeam and Harris, 2004).

The theory guiding practice in health promotion is not yet well developed. The theories concerning psycho-social determinants of health in individuals are the least complex and best tested according to traditional criteria. The different theories and models which may be useful to guide elements of programmes directed to community mobilization and organizational change are generally less well formed and far less amenable to testing through typical experimental research designs. However, the importance of community mobilization and organizational and policy change for health is so great that it is essential to identify and apply our best current understanding of these issues.

There is no single theory or model that can adequately guide the development of a comprehensive health promotion programme intended to influence the multiple determinants of health in populations (see Table 3.1 in Chapter 3). Practitioners need to use local knowledge and experience, in addition to available research information, to make judgements about community needs and the determinants of health that are most amenable to change at any particular time. In developing a comprehensive strategy to tackle a defined health priority, practitioners will be assisted by making judicious use of theories and models. Multi-level interventions will generally be more powerful than single-track programmes. Correspondingly, programmes will need to draw on several theories and models in the development of a comprehensive strategy. If applied wisely, these theories will help guide decisions, may predict the likely outcomes, and help explain the reasons for success.

Not all practitioners have the position or capacity to operate at multiple levels. In such cases, a knowledge of theories will help practitioners to maximize the potential effectiveness of their interventions, and to place into perspective their efforts alongside the range of opportunities for action.

Theory of innovation diffusion

The systematic study of the ways in which new ideas are adopted by communities led to the development of the *theory of innovation diffusion* (Rogers, 2002). It is based on the idea that there are five factors that influence the success and speed with which new ideas are adopted in communities. Understanding these factors is central to the application of diffusion theory to health promotion. The factors are:

- the characteristics of the potential adopters
- the rate of adoption
- the nature of the social system

- the characteristics of the innovation
- the characteristics of change agents

A widely used system of categorizing adopters is based on the time it takes for adoption to occur. This identifies *innovators* as those 2–3 per cent of the population who are quickest to adopt new ideas, and *early adopters* as the 10–15 per cent of the population who may be more mainstream within the community but are the most amenable to change and have some of the personal, social or financial resources to adopt the innovation. The *early majority* are the 30–35 per cent of the population who are amenable to change, and have become persuaded of the benefits of adopting the innovation. The *late majority* are the 30–35 per cent of the population who are sceptics and are reluctant to adopt new ideas until such time as the benefits have been clearly established. And, finally, the *laggards* are the 10–20 per cent of the population who are seen to be the most conservative and in many cases actively resistant to the introduction of new ideas. As indicated by the different percentages for each group, Rogers suggests that their distribution in a population matches the 'normal' probability distribution curve.

From this simple classification it is possible to see how age, disposable income and exposure to the media, for example, are important variables which will define the different types of 'adopter' and influence the speed of uptake of innovations. Some innovations take much longer than others to introduce to the majority of the target population and, in some cases, will never reach the entire population. The increasing difficulty of influencing late adopters and the residual group of laggards translates into diminishing returns on effort in health promotion programmes and needs to be recognized in the planning and evaluation of such programmes.

Analysis of programmes has led to the identification of *characteristics of innovations* that have been consistently associated with successful adoption. These include:

- *Compatibility* with prevailing socio-economic and cultural values of the adopter. For example, if a change in diet is being advocated in a particular community, it is more likely to be adopted if the food is based on traditional food sources.
- Clarity of the *relative advantage* of the innovation compared with current practices, including *perceived cost-effectiveness*, as well as usefulness, convenience and prestige. For example, is the food (such as fresh fruit and vegetables) conveniently available at a price that people can afford.
- The *simplicity and flexibility* of the innovation. Those which require simple actions and which can be adapted to different circumstances are more likely to be successful. For example, is the food simple to prepare and consume, and are any new cooking methods required.
- The *reversibility and perceived risk* of adoption. Innovations perceived as high risk or involving an irreversible change in practice are less likely to be adopted. For example, no new cooking utensils need to be bought.
- *Observability* of the results of adopting an innovation to others who may be contemplating change. For example, there are stories in local news media showing the impact of a changed diet on a person's life.

Finally, Rogers identifies the importance of the *change agent* – the person who facilitates the adoption of change in a population. This may be an external person working with a community to introduce an innovation or may be a person from within the community. Allied to this, community members can act *as role models* for other adopters. Selection of appropriate role models, particularly from among community leaders, can help accelerate the rate of adoption in a community.

Diffusion of innovation theory provides guidance on how to introduce new health behaviour into a community. It helps health promotion workers to define what it is they are intending to achieve and provides practical guidance on how this can be done. It also helps you to think about why, how and in what way local communities may be involved in health promotion programmes.

 Activity 4.1

You have been asked to develop a programme to promote condom use in your community. Use the *characteristics of innovations* from the *diffusion of innovation theory* to help you to decide on factors that might be associated with a greater chance of success.

 Feedback

The answer will be different depending on the country or community you are thinking of. However, you should have considered:

1 *Compatibility* of condom use with the cultural values and socio-economic climate of the people you are asking to change (i.e. the 'adopters'). Different values and taboos are associated with condom use.

2 *Relative advantage* of using condoms compared with current practices – that is, the costs and benefits to people of using condoms. You should also have considered the availability and affordability.

3 *Simplicity and flexibility* of what you are asking people. This may sound easy or simple but in practice negotiating condom use is extremely difficult for many.

4 *Reversibility and perceived risk* of adoption. In the example of condom use, perceived risk is likely to be more of an issue; you are asking people to put themselves in a potentially embarrassing situation, where the risk might be to their self-esteem or reputation.

5 *Observability* – can others see the benefits of adopting the behaviour?

The communication-behaviour change model

Effective health promotion strategies are best developed by engaging individuals and communities in the issue to be addressed. This involves understanding the beliefs and knowledge that people have about a problem and their skills in addressing it, as well as broader community understanding of why the issue is important and how it can most effectively be tackled.

Clear communication between health promotion practitioners and those whom they are trying to influence is essential. The *communication-behaviour change model* was developed by McGuire (1989) to design and guide public education campaigns. It is included here because the model is based on communication *inputs* and *outputs* that are designed to influence attitudes and behaviour in similar ways to the theories and models described in Chapter 3.

The five communication *inputs* described by McGuire are:

1 *Source:* the person, group or organization from whom a message is perceived to have come. The source can influence the credibility, clarity and relevance of a message. For example, the same message delivered from a government source, by a celebrity or from a non-governmental organization will have different credibility and relevance to different target audiences
2 *Message:* what is said and how it is said. The content and form of a message can influence audience response. For example, the use of fear or humour to communicate the same message may provoke different responses from different target audiences. Practical considerations such as the length of the message, form of language and tone of voice also need to be considered.
3 *Channel:* the medium through which a message is delivered. Mass media include television, radio and print media (e.g. newspapers, pamphlets, posters), as well as techniques such as direct mail. More recently, information technology has opened up a range of new media for use in communicating health messages in high-income countries, including the internet and mobile phone text messages. Issues to be considered in selecting a channel for communication include the potential reach of different media, the cost of use, and differences in the complexity of message which can be communicated through different media.
4 *Receiver:* the intended target audience. Recognizing differences in audience segments and their media preferences are important in matching the right message to the right channel from the right source. Social and demographic variables such as gender, age, ethnicity, income and location, as well as current attitudes and behaviours, and media use can all be considered as a part of this element.
5 *Destination:* the desired outcome to the communication. This may include change in attitudes or beliefs, or, more likely, changes in behaviour.

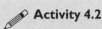 **Activity 4.2**

This model can be very useful in conceptualizing and designing mass communication strategies. Try highlighting a men's health issue such as the risk of prostate cancer.

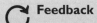 **Feedback**

It will be important for the source of the message to be someone respected by the men most at risk and with whom they can identify. The message will need to be portrayed in an acceptable way, for example by using humour to portray situations men face. It will need to be communicated through media used by these men, with decisions made on which messages can best be communicated by TV, which by printed material and which through advertisements. There will need to be some decision on who is the target group: Is it all men? What are the subgroups? How influential are 'significant others', such as partners and parents, in bringing about change? And, finally, what is it that the communication strategy is hoping to achieve: awareness raising, or some more specific action?

The communication-behaviour change model also provides a twelve-step sequence of events, representing *outputs* from a communication, which link initial exposure to a communication to long-term change in behaviour. This model illustrates that for a communication strategy to be effective, the message has to be carefully designed and delivered through an appropriate channel to reach the target audience. The population has to be exposed to the message (no mean feat in itself!), pay attention to it and understand it. Once understood by an individual, the message must create an inclination to change, reflected in attitude change which is stored and maintained until such time as the recipient is in a position to act on that attitude change. Once the decision to change a behaviour has been made and acted on, this new behaviour needs reinforcement to be maintained.

These inputs and outputs can be put together as a matrix to illustrate the need to change the input mix depending on the targeted output. Different sources, messages and channels will be required to reach different people and achieve different outcomes.

The communication-behaviour change model shows just how difficult it can be to develop a public communication campaign which by itself leads to sustainable behaviour change. This model provides an excellent overview of the range of issues that need to be considered in the development of a public education campaign. Although several major public intervention programmes (such as the first Stanford three-cities programme in the USA, which was intended to reduce the risks for heart disease in the community) have been based on this model, progressive experience in using the mass media for public communication has led to a better understanding of the advantages and limitations of media campaigns in terms of cost, reach and effect. Media campaigns are now more commonly used to influence public knowledge, attitudes and opinions as a part of a more comprehensive strategy that places mass communication within a wider repertoire of interventions.

Activity 4.3

What key messages and planning steps would you need if you were responsible for the implementation of a new immunization programme? Take account of the individual health behaviour change models, the diffusion of innovations through communities and the attention to communication. Think either of introducing a new immunization in high-income countries and bear in mind the concerns that have been brought to the fore with the issues over MMR (measles, mumps and rubella) vaccine, or introducing a previously unavailable vaccine in a low-income country.

Feedback

Your plan should reflect not only an understanding of the individual characteristics explained by the health belief model and stages of change, but also a broader recognition of the knowledge and understanding in the community as a whole, the difference between individual and mass media messages, and the attention to the steps in the process and the roles of various agents, both professional and community.

Model of organizational change

Health promotion practitioners are interested in influencing organizations for several reasons:

- people are usually employed by organizations and have an interest in ensuring that their own organization is able to support the work that we are doing
- people are interested in influencing the activities or policies of other organizations who have an influence on the health of the population
- you have to find ways to enable organizations to work together to promote the health of the population.

Goodman *et al.* (2002) have succinctly described the problems and potential rewards of facilitating change in organizations:

Organisations are layered. Their strata range from the surrounding environment at the broadest level, to the overall organisational structure, to the management within, to work groups, to each individual member. Change may be influenced at each of these strata, and health promotion strategies that are directed at several layers simultaneously may be most durable in producing the desired results. The health professional who understands the ecology of organisations and who can apply appropriate strategies has a powerful tool for change.

Unlike many of the theories and models described above, the application of theories of organizational change is far less developed and tested.

Four stages of the model

Goodman and colleagues (2002) propose a four-stage model for organizational change that is applicable to health promotion. They emphasize the importance of recognizing the different stages and of matching strategies to promote change in each of the stages, similar in structure to the stages of the two models you have already encountered in this chapter.

In the model, Stage 1 is described as *awareness raising*. This stage is intended to stimulate interest and support for organizational change at a senior level by clarifying health problems in the organizational environment, and identifying potential solutions. For example, awareness raising may involve senior managers and administrators in the education system becoming concerned about tobacco control and recognizing the potential role to be played by the education system. These senior administrators are likely to be the most influential in decisions to adopt new policies and programmes in an organization. If they are convinced of the importance of a problem and the need for a solution involving their organization, then the strategy moves to the next stage.

Stage 2 is described as *adoption* and involves planning for and adoption of a policy, programme or other innovation that addresses the problem identified in Stage 1. This includes the identification of resources necessary for implementation. In larger organizations, this stage will often involve a different level in the management structure – the gatekeepers – who are more closely associated with the day-to-day running of an organization. In the example, this could involve school principals and senior teachers responsible for school curricula and organization.

Ideally, this stage will involve negotiation and adaptation of intervention ideas to make them compatible with the circumstances of individual organizations. This element of *adaptation* is often essential to the adoption of change in organizations, but is frequently missed by those attempting to disseminate new ideas through organizations.

Stage 3 is described as *implementation* and is concerned with technical aspects of programme delivery, including the provision of training and material support needed for the introduction of change. In the example, this could involve class-room teachers, as they will be most directly responsible for the introduction of change. This phase may involve training and the provision of resource support to foster the successful introduction of a programme. This *capacity building* is essential for the successful introduction and maintenance of change in organizations. Many policy initiatives fail at this point because too little attention is given to the detail of the implementation process and too little support is offered to the individuals at the level at which implementation takes place.

Stage 4 is described as *institutionalization* and is concerned with the long-term maintenance of an innovation, once it has been successfully introduced. Senior administrators again become the leading players, by establishing systems for monitoring and quality control, including continued investment in resources and training.

Organizational climate, culture and capacity

In developing their ideas, Goodman and colleagues (2002) drew upon several established theories that describe and explain organizational change and development. These theories have evolved to include environmental influences and how the norms of entire organizations are transformed. The related concepts of organizational climate, organizational culture and organizational capacity need to be recognized and understood in the execution of a staged approach to organizational change described above.

Organizational climate is often referred to as the 'personality' of an organization. It refers to those characteristics that distinguish one organization from another, based on the collective perceptions of those who live and work in that environment and who influence their behaviour. For example, some schools are more or less authoritarian in their relations with students; public services are more or less customer focused; some work sites value and reward staff loyalty more than others. These characteristics are seen as dynamic and are affected by a wide range of variables, many of which are external to the organization. The term *organizational culture* is often used interchangeably with climate, but is distinguished as meaning a set of values and assumptions about an organization that have formed over time, are more stable and resistant to change. Both organizational climate and culture can influence an organization's capacity to function effectively, and in turn may determine the outcome of efforts to bring about change in organizations. *Organizational capacity* can also be seen in more practical terms, such as having appropriately trained personnel, effective management systems and sufficient resources. Organizational climate, culture and capacity are all important variables that will influence the pace and extent of change that may be achieved through the stage process described above.

Achieving organizational change may involve interventions designed to alter the organizational climate and to build organizational capacity. *Capacity building* is an important element of effective health promotion. Hawe and colleagues (1997) have defined capacity building as 'the development of sustainable skills, structures, resources and commitment to health improvement . . . to prolong and multiply health gains many times over'. It is sometimes described as the invisible work of health promotion. It includes activities as diverse as canvassing the opportunities for a programme, lobbying for support, developing skills, supporting policy development, negotiating with management, developing partnerships and making organizational plans.

The importance of focusing on organizations

The model of organizational change provides useful guidance on the different steps required to introduce and sustain a programme in different organizational settings. In particular, it highlights:

- the need to *understand the core business* of an organization, and its *organizational structure*, determine how a health promotion programme can fit within these parameters, and help to achieve the core business goals
- the need to work with individuals at *different levels* in an organization as well as between organizations
- the inherently political nature of the task of *influencing senior managers*
- the importance of *flexibility in negotiation* with 'gatekeepers' concerning the adoption of a programme
- the need to support those individuals responsible for the delivery of a programme or innovation
- the need to establish a *system for longer term maintenance* and quality control.

One of the major reasons that the health sector is interested in working with organizations is to bring about systematic and lasting change that will address some of the basic determinants of health, such as safe workplaces, improved living conditions and the development of recreational facilities. Understanding how to do this most effectively has the potential to have profound impacts on health.

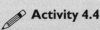 **Activity 4.4**

Reflect on the plan you produced for Activity 4.3.

1 While you may have considered the roles of organizations in your plan, is there anything you would add now having considered the model of organizational change?
2 How much more complex would it be if you were aiming to change long-term socially determined behaviours rather than some simple behaviour?

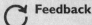 **Feedback**

1 You should have considered the role of senior managers and those who set the policies for your organization and how you will raise their awareness of the issues. This may have two perspectives: what should be done for employees of the organization, or what role can the organization have in promoting a health behaviour change.

Once there is an understanding of the issues, a plan for how change will be adopted is needed. You should have considered who would need to be involved in this process and this would be both top down (managerial commitment) and bottom up (workforce and public inputs).

Implementation of the plan may require a programme of staff training and support being given to those in the organization who will have to change their behaviour. This is likely to be required until the change in behaviour has become the organizational norm and become institutionalized.

2 In terms of increasing the uptake of immunization, there is a clear and measurable outcome to the change. In your consideration of the wider health issues for an organization, you might have looked at a range of possible policy areas. For example, how to increase physical activity or healthy eating, how to reduce smoking, or how to make working practices healthier. In each case, this would involve participation by a range of policy makers in the organization, as well as require commitment to the change by staff.

Summary

You have seen how theories and models can help you to conceive and plan health promotion programmes at the community and organizational levels. In particular, you have learnt about the theory of innovation diffusion, of communication behaviour change and of organizational change. In the next section, you will learn about some of the practical considerations that must be taken into account when applying these theories and models.

References

Goodman RM, Steckler A, Kegler MC (2002) Mobilising organisations for health enhancement: theories of organisational change, in Glanz K et al (eds.) Health behaviour and health education: theory, research and practice. San Francisco: Jossey-Bass

Hawe P, Noort M, King L, Jorden C (1997). Multiplying health gains: the critical role of capacity building in health promotion programs. Health Policy 39: 29–42

McGuire WJ (1989) Theoretical foundations of campaigns, in Rice RE and Atkin C (eds.) *Public Communication Campaigns*. Thousand Oaks, CA: Sage

Nutbeam D, Harris E (2004) *Theory in a Nutshell: A Practical Guide to Health Promotion Theories*. Sydney, NSW: McGraw-Hill

Rogers EM (2002) Diffusion of preventive interventions. Addictive Behaviours 27: 989–93

SECTION 2

Epidemiology, politics and ethics

Determinants of health

Overview

In this chapter you will learn about the range of factors that have an impact on the ability of individuals, communities and societies to develop and maintain good health and well-being. It highlights the importance of the social determinants of health and discusses issues relating to the measurement of socio-economic status, definitions of health inequalities and the issues that need to be addressed if health inequalities are to be reduced.

Learning objectives

After working through this chapter, you will be better able to:

- describe the major influences on health
- understand the relationship between health and socio-economic status
- compare the four different explanations for socio-economic inequalities in health
- understand the challenges of addressing health inequalities

Key terms

Inequalities in health Differences in health status between different population sub-groups.

Social classes Categories based on the occupation of the head of a household.

Social inequities Differences in opportunity for different population sub-groups.

What determines health?

It is recognized that the health and well-being of people is influenced by a range of factors, both within and outside the individual's control (Lalonde, 1974; WHO, 1998). This has led to the development of a number of models that attempt to identify the determinants of health and the pathways through which they operate. One such model frequently used in international and national policy documents is Dahlgren and Whitehead's (1991) 'Policy Rainbow', which describes the layers of influence on an individual's potential for health (Figure 5.1). They describe factors which are fixed (such as age, sex and genetic) and factors which are potentially modifiable, expressed as a series of layers of influence, including individual lifestyle

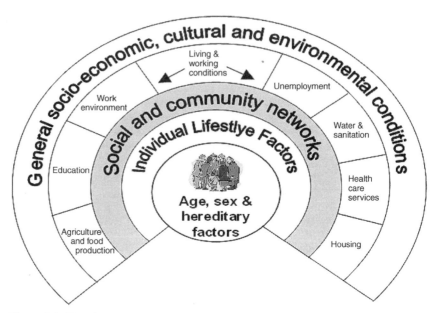

Figure 5.1 The policy rainbow
Source: Dahlgren and Whitehead (1991)

factors, social and community networks, and general socio-economic, cultural and environmental conditions.

The model of Dahlgren and Whitehead has been useful in providing a framework for raising questions about the size of the contribution of each of the layers to health, the feasibility of changing specific factors and the complementary action that would be required to influence factors in other layers. It has helped researchers to construct a range of hypotheses about the determinants of health, to explore the relative influence of these determinants on health and the interactions between the various determinants.

Over the last thirty years, researchers from different disciplines have explained the relative importance of the range of determinants on health and how they impact on different sectors of society. Some examples include:

- Marmot *et al.* (1978) demonstrated gradients in mortality across grades of employment among English civil servants.
- Bartley *et al.* (1994) have shown that children and adolescents living in poorer quality housing are more likely to have been of low birth weight.
- Townsend *et al.* (1988) have shown that material deprivation (e.g. overcrowding, housing tenure, unemployment) is a predictor of mortality and limiting long-term illness.
- Barker (1998) has shown that the *in utero* experience is linked to the risk of developing diseases later in life.
- Graham (2001) has demonstrated the cumulative effect of social disadvantage over the life course and the contribution of poor early life circumstances.

- McGinnis *et al.* (2002) have demonstrated the relative impact that various health determinants make on mortality in the USA: 30 per cent due to genetic predispositions, 15 per cent due to social circumstances, 5 per cent due to environmental exposures, 40 per cent due to behavioural patterns and 10 per cent due to shortfalls in health care.

Such findings may help policy makers decide where investments should be made to achieve the greatest impact on promoting health. However, McGinnis and colleagues (2002) were keen to highlight that more important than the proportions is the nature of the influences in play where the determinants intersect. For example, genetic predisposition is influenced by environmental exposures and behavioural choices made by parents; the nature and consequences of behavioural choices are affected by social circumstances and social circumstances affect the health care people receive.

While each of the determinants is important in its own right, health is determined at every stage of life, by complex interactions between social and economic factors, the physical environment and individual behaviour.

Activity 5.1

The Lalonde Report (1974) was one of the first publications to document the major influences on health and to identify the courses of action that needed to be taken if health improvements were to be made. The following extracts describe the 'Health Field Concept'. As you read them, prepare answers to the following questions:

1 What are the main influences on health status and what is their relative importance?
2 What is the Health Field Concept and how has it been useful to advance the health of Canadians?
3 What dangers do you perceive in this sort of approach?

 ## The Health Field Concept

A basic problem in analysing the health field has been the absence of an agreed conceptual framework for sub-dividing it into its principal elements. Without such a framework, it has been difficult to communicate properly or to break up the field into manageable segments, amenable to analysis and evaluation. It was felt keenly that there was a need to organize the thousands of pieces into an orderly pattern that was both intellectually acceptable and sufficiently simple to permit the quick location, in the pattern, of almost any idea, problem or activity related to health: a sort of map of the health territory.

Such a Health Field Concept was developed during the preparation of this paper. It envisages that the health field can be broken up into four broad elements: HUMAN BIOLOGY, ENVIRONMENT, LIFESTYLE and HEALTH CARE ORGANIZATION. These four elements were identified through an examination of the causes and underlying factors of sickness and death in Canada and from an assessment of the parts these elements play in affecting the level of health in Canada.

Human Biology

The HUMAN BIOLOGY element includes all those aspects of health, both physical and mental, which are developed within the human body as a consequence of the basic biology of man and the organic make-up of the individual. This element includes the genetic inheritance of the individual, the processes of maturation and aging, and the body's many complex internal systems, such as skeletal, nervous, muscular, cardio-vascular, endocrine, digestive and so on. As the human body is such a complicated organism, the health implications of human biology are numerous, varied and serious and the things that can go wrong with it are legion. Health problems originating from human biology are causing untold miseries and costing billions of dollars in treatment services.

Environment

The ENVIRONMENT category includes all those matters related to health which are external to the human body and over which the individual has little or no control. Individuals cannot, by themselves, ensure that foods, drugs, cosmetics, devices, water supply, etc. are safe and uncontaminated; that the health hazards of air, water and noise pollution are controlled; that the spread of communicable diseases is prevented; that effective garbage and sewage disposal is carried out; and that the social environment, including the rapid changes in it, do not have harmful effects on health.

Lifestyle

The LIFESTYLE category, in the Health Field Concept, consists of the aggregation of decisions by individuals which affect their health and over which they more or less have control . . . Personal decisions and habits that are bad, from a health point of view, creating self-imposed risks. When those risks result in illness or death, the victim's lifestyle can be said to have contributed to, or caused, this.

Health care organization

The fourth category in the concept is HEALTH CARE ORGANIZATION, which consists of the quantity, quality, arrangement, nature and relationships of people and resources in the provision of health care . . . Until now most of society's efforts to improve health, and the bulk of direct health expenditures, have been focused on HEALTH CARE ORGANIZATION. Yet, when we identify the present main causes of sickness and death in Canada, we find that they are rooted in the other three elements of the Concept: HUMAN BIOLOGY, ENVIRONMENT and LIFESTYLE. It is apparent, therefore, that vast sums are being spent treating diseases that could have been prevented in the first place. Greater attention to the first three conceptual elements is needed if we are to continue to reduce disability and early death.

Characteristics of the health field concept

The HEALTH FIELD CONCEPT has many characteristics which make it a powerful tool for analysing health problems, determining the health needs of Canadians and choosing the means by which those needs can be met. One of the evident consequences of the Health Field Concept has been to raise HUMAN BIOLOGY, ENVIRONMENT and LIFESTYLE to a level of categorical importance, equal to that of HEALTH CARE ORGANIZATION. This, in itself, is a radical step in view of the clear pre-eminence that HEALTH CARE ORGANIZATION has had in past concepts of the health field. A second attribute of the Concept is that it is comprehensive. Any health problem can be traced to one, or a combination of, the four elements. This comprehensiveness is important because it ensures that all aspects of health will be given due consideration and that all who

contribute to health, individually and collectively – patient, physician, scientist and government – are aware of their roles and their influence on the level of health. A third feature is
that the Concept permits a system of analysis by which any question can be examined
under the four elements in order to assess their relative significance and interaction. For
example, the underlying causes of death from traffic accidents can be found to be due
mainly to risks taken by individuals, with lesser importance given to the design of cars and
roads, and to the availability of emergency treatment. Human biology has little or no
significance in this area. In order of importance, therefore, LIFESTYLE, ENVIRONMENT
and HEALTH CARE ORGANIZATION contribute to traffic deaths in the proportions of
something like 75%, 20% and 5% respectively.

This analysis permits programme planners to focus their attention on the most important
contributing factors. Similar assessments of the relative importance of contributing factors
can be made for many other health problems. A fourth feature of the Concept is that it
permits a further sub-division of factors. Again, for traffic deaths in the Lifestyle category,
the risks taken by individuals can be classed under impaired driving, carelessness, failure to
wear seat-belts and speeding. In many ways the Concept thus provides a roadmap which
shows the most direct links between health problems, and their underlying causes, and the
relative importance of various contributing factors. Finally, the Health Field Concept provides a new perspective on health, a perspective which frees creative minds for the recognition and exploration of hitherto neglected fields. The importance for their own health of
the behaviour and habits of individual Canadians is an example of the kind of conclusion
that is obtainable by using the Health Field Concept as an analytical tool.

One of the main problems in improving the health of Canadians is that the essential power
to do so is widely dispersed among individual citizens, governments, health professions and
institutions. This fragmentation of responsibility has sometimes led to imbalanced
approaches, with each participant in the health field pursuing solutions only within his area
of interest. Under the Health Field Concept, the fragments are brought together into a
unified whole which permits everyone to see the importance of all factors, including those
which are the responsibility of others. This unified view of the health field may well turn
out to be one of the Concept's main contributions to progress in improving the level of
health.

Issues arising from the use of the health field concept
The Concept was designed with two aims in view: to provide a greater understanding of
what contributes to sickness and death, and to facilitate the identification of courses of
action that might be taken to improve health. The Concept is *not* an organizational framework for structuring programmes and activities to one or another of the four elements of
the Concept would be contrary to reality and would perpetuate the present fragmentary
approach to solving health problems. For example, the problem of drug abuse needs
attention by researchers in human biology, by behavioural scientists, by those who adminis-
ter drug laws and by those who provide personal health care. Contributions are necessary
from all of these and it would be a misuse of the Health Field Concept to exploit it as a
basis for capturing all aspects of a problem for one particular unit of organization, or
interest group . . .

[Another] issue, more theoretical, was whether or not it was possible to divide external
influences on health between the environment, about which the individual can do little, and
lifestyle, in which he can make choices. Particularly cogent were arguments that personal

choices were dictated by environmental factors, such as the peer-group pressures to start smoking cigarettes during the teens. Further, it was argued that some bad personal habits were so ingrained as to constitute addictions which, by definition, no longer permitted a choice by a simple act of will. Smoking, alcohol abuse and drug abuse were some of the lifestyle problems referred to in this vein. The fact that there is some truth in both hypotheses, i.e. that environment affects lifestyle and that some personal habits are addictive, requires a philosophical and moral response, rather than a purely intellectual one. This response is that if we simply give up on individuals whose lifestyles create excessive risks to their health, we will be abandoning those who could have changed, and will be perpetuating the very environment which influenced them adversely in the first place. In short, the deterministic view must be put aside in favour of faith in the power of free will, hobbled as this power may be at times by environment and addiction.

One point on which no quarter can be given is that difficulties in categorizing the contributing factors to a given health problem are no excuse for putting the problem aside. The problem does not disappear because of difficulties in fitting it nicely into a conceptual framework. Another issue is whether or not the Concept will be used to carry too much of an analytical workload, by demanding that it serve both to identify requirements for health and to determine the mechanisms for meeting them. Although the Concept will help bring out the problems and their causes and even point to the avenues by which they can be solved, it cannot determine the precise steps that are needed to implement programmes. Decisions as to programmes are affected by so many other considerations that they will require the analysis of many practical factors outside the Concept proper.

The ultimate philosophical issue raised by the Concept is whether, and to what extent, government can get into the business of modifying human behaviour, even if it does so to improve health. The marketing of social change is a new field which applies the marketing techniques of the business world to getting people to change their behaviour, i.e. eating habits, exercise habits, smoking habits, driving habits, etc. It is argued by some that proficiency in social marketing would inevitably lead governments into all kinds of undesirable thought control and propaganda. The dangers of governmental proficiency in social marketing are recognized, but so are the evident abuses resulting from all other kinds of marketing. If the siren song of coloured television, for example, is creating an indolent and passive use of leisure time, has the government not the duty to counteract its effects by marketing programmes aimed at promoting physical recreation? As previously mentioned, in Canada some 76% of the population over age 13 devotes less than one hour a week to participation in sports, while 84% of the same population spends four or more hours weekly watching television. This kind of imbalance extends to the amount of money being spent by the private sector on marketing products and services, some of which if abused, contribute to sickness and death. One must inevitably conclude that society, through government, owes it to itself to develop protective marketing techniques to counteract those abuses.

Finally, some have questioned whether an increased emphasis on human biology, environment and lifestyle will not lead to a diminution of attention to the system of personal health care. This issue is raised particularly by those whose activities are centred on the health care organization. On this issue it can be said, that Canadians would not tolerate a reduction in personal health care and are in fact pushing very hard to make services more accessible and more comprehensive . . .

More important, if the incidence of sickness can be reduced by prevention then the cost of present services will go down, or at least the rate of increase will diminish. This will make money available to extend health insurance to more and more services and to provide needed facilities, such as ambulatory care centres and extended care institutions. To a considerable extent, therefore, the increased availability of health care services to Canadians depends upon the success that can be achieved in preventing illness through measures taken in human biology, environment and lifestyle.

 Feedback

1 The main influences on health status are: human biology, environment, lifestyle and health care organization. Their relative importance varies according to the health problem. For example, congenital anomalies will largely be due to human biology and the environment, whereas coronary heart disease will be determined by all four categories.

2 The health field concept provides a framework to ensure that all four categories of determinants are considered when a health problem is being addressed by policy makers. It has been useful in shifting the balance of attention from personal health care to the promotion of health through environmental measures and attempts to change people's lifestyles.

3 The main danger is that knowledge of the determinants of illness and disease is inevitably limited and conditional. For example, although written only thirty years ago, most people working to prevent road accidents would now emphasize the importance of the environment over the lifestyle factors that Lalonde focused on.

The importance of the social determinants of health

Research efforts over the last thirty years have documented how health is socially patterned (Townsend *et al.*, 1988; Harris *et al.*, 1999). Health status is influenced by individual characteristics and behaviour (lifestyles) but continues to be significantly determined by the different social, economic and environmental circumstances of individuals and populations. Disease prevalence, life expectancy, behavioural risk factors and general well-being all display social gradients related to socio-economic status as well as sex, age and ethnicity. In other words, people living in different socio-economic environments face different risks of ill health and death. In general, the least affluent have much poorer health than the most affluent. For example:

- In the Netherlands, men with higher educational attainment have 12.6 more healthy years of life than those with lower educational levels
- In England, death from coronary heart disease is higher among unskilled men than those in professional groups
- In Finland, men with the highest educational attainment have 13 more disability-free years than those with the lowest attainment, but the difference is only eight years for women

The World Health Organization brought together some of the most influential research in this area in 2003. They concluded that:

> even in the most affluent countries, people who are less well off have substantially shorter life expectancies and more illnesses than the rich. Not only are these differences in health an important social injustice, they have also drawn scientific attention to some of the most powerful determinants of health standards in modern societies. They have led in particular to a growing understanding of the remarkable sensitivity of health to the social environment and to what have become known as the social determinants of health.

The report presents what is known about the relationship between the social determinants and health and highlights the policy implications. Table 5.1 presents the ten topics covered in the report, to illustrate the importance of the social determinants of health.

Table 5.1 Ten major social determinants of health

Topic	Summary statement
Social gradient	Life expectancy is shorter and most diseases are more common further down the social ladder in each society
Stress	Stressful circumstances, making people feel worried, anxious and unable to cope, are damaging to health and may lead to premature death
Early life	A good start in life means supporting mothers and young children: the health impact of early development and education lasts a lifetime
Social exclusion	Life is short where its quality is poor. By causing hardship and resentment, poverty, social exclusion and discrimination cost lives
Work	Stress in the workplace increases the risk of disease. People who have more control over their work have better health
Unemployment	Job security increases health, well-being and job satisfaction. Higher rates of unemployment cause more illness and premature death
Social support	Friendship, good social relations and strong supportive networks improve health at home, at work and in the community
Addiction	Individuals turn to alcohol, drugs and tobacco and suffer from their use, but use is influenced by the wider social setting
Food	Because global market forces control the food supply, healthy food is a political issue
Transport	Healthy transport means less driving and more walking and cycling, backed up by better public transport

Source: WHO (2003)

The intention of the WHO report was to ensure that policy at all levels – government, public and private institutions, workplaces and the community – takes proper account of evidence suggesting a wide responsibility for creating healthy societies. The following is taken from the introduction to the report.

The solid facts

Health policy was once thought to be about little more than the provision and funding of medical care: the social determinants of health were discussed only among academics. This is now changing. While medical care can prolong survival and improve prognosis after some serious diseases, more important for the health of the population as a whole are the social and economic conditions that make people ill and in need of medical care in the first place.

Nevertheless, universal access to medical care is clearly one of the social determinants of health. Why also, in a new publication on the determinants of health, is there nothing about genes? The new discoveries on the human genome are exciting in the promise they hold for advances in the understanding and treatment of specific diseases. But however important *individual* genetic susceptibilities to disease may be, the common causes of the ill health that affects *populations* are environmental: they come and go far more quickly than the slow pace of genetic change because they reflect the changes in the way we live. This is why life expectancy has improved so dramatically over recent generations; it is also why some European countries have improved their health while others have not, and it is why health differences between different social groups have widened or narrowed as social and economic conditions have changed. The evidence on which this publication is based comes from very large numbers of research reports – many thousands in all. Some of the studies have used prospective methods, sometimes following tens of thousands of people over decades – sometimes from birth. Others have used cross-sectional methods and have studied individual, area, national or international data. Difficulties that have sometimes arisen (perhaps despite follow-up studies) in determining causality have been overcome by using evidence from intervention studies, from so-called natural experiments, and occasionally from studies of other primate species.

Nevertheless, as both health and the major influences on it vary substantially according to levels of economic development, the reader should keep in mind that the bulk of the evidence on which this publication is based comes from rich developed countries and its relevance to less developed countries may be limited. Our intention has been to ensure that policy at all levels – in government, public and private institutions, workplaces and the community – takes proper account of recent evidence suggesting a wider responsibility for creating healthy societies.

But a publication as short as this cannot provide a comprehensive guide to determinants of public health. Several areas of health policy, such as the need to safeguard people from exposure to toxic materials at work, are left out because they are well known (though often not adequately enforced). As exhortations to individual behaviour change are also a well established approach to health promotion, and the evidence suggests they may sometimes have limited effect, there is little about what individuals can do to improve their own health. We do, however, emphasize the need to understand how behaviour is shaped by the environment and, consistent with approaching health through its social determinants, recommend environmental changes that would lead to healthier behaviour.

Given that this publication was put together from the contributions of acknowledged experts in each field, what is striking is the extent to which the sections converge on the need for a more just and caring society – both economically and socially. Combining economics, sociology and psychology with neurobiology and medicine, it looks as if much depends on understanding the interaction between material disadvantage and its social meanings. It is not simply that poor material circumstances are harmful to health; the social meaning of being poor, unemployed, socially excluded, or otherwise stigmatized also matters. As social beings, we need not only good material conditions but, from early childhood onwards, we need to feel valued and appreciated. We need friends, we need more sociable societies, we need to feel useful, and we need to exercise a significant degree of control over meaningful work. Without these we become more prone to depression, drug use, anxiety, hostility and feelings of hopelessness, which all rebound on physical health. We hope that by tackling some of the material and social injustices, policy will not only improve health and well-being, but may also reduce a range of other social problems that flourish alongside ill health and are rooted in some of the same socioeconomic processes.

 Activity 5.2

1   How does this report define the social determinants of health?
2   What are the specific actions required of policy makers to take account of the social determinants?
3   Compare the definitions used in this report with the ones used by Lalonde, White-head and McGinnis. How consistent are they in defining the social determinants of health?
4   What are the main causes of inequalities in health as described in this report?

 Feedback

1   Social determinants of health are defined in terms of environmental factors, such as exposure to toxic materials at work, economic factors and social factors, such as exercising a degree of control over meaningful work.

2   Policy makers are required to recognize the social determinants and accept that the responsibility for creating a healthy society requires more than good quality personal health care.

3   The definitions used in all sources are consistent. They all recognize four principal causes of ill health: biology (including genetics), the environment, lifestyle (personal behaviour) and health care.

4   The main causes of inequalities in health identified in the WHO report are environmental, both the physical and the socio-economic environment.

Understanding health inequalities

As you have seen, inequalities in health exist in all countries and since the 1950s these inequalities have been increasing in some countries despite improvements in welfare provision. This suggests that while health policies, interventions and initiatives have led to an overall improvement in health, they have failed some segments of our societies.

There is debate in the scientific literature about the difference between health inequalities and health inequities. The following definitions are helpful in distinguishing between the two:

- *Health inequality* describes differences in health between different population groups – according to socio-economic status, geographical area, age, disability, sex or ethnicity.
- *Health inequity* describes differences in opportunity for different population groups which result in unequal access to health services, nutritious food, adequate housing, etc. These can lead to health inequalities.

At an international level, the World Health Organization has shown its commitment to support action on inequalities in its Health21 strategy (WHO, 1998), in which its target is to reduce the health gap between socio-economic groups within countries by at least a quarter in all member states by substantially improving the health of disadvantaged groups.

At a national level, there is a growing number of examples of governments developing comprehensive strategies, programmes and initiatives to tackle inequalities. One example in the UK is Tackling Health Inequalities: A Programme for Action (Department of Health, 2003) which identifies the need to address the wider influences on health by taking action in a number of key areas:

- reducing levels of child poverty
- improving the quality of poor housing
- improving the accessibility, punctuality, reliability and use of local transport
- improving educational attainment and tackling low basic skills
- tackling worklessness and inactivity
- strengthening disadvantaged communities through improving access to social and community facilities and services

Getting inequalities on the agenda of governments is one step in the right direction to provide equal opportunities for everyone in society to maintain good health. However, Graham (2004) argues that government strategies will only be effective in tackling health inequalities if they are able to make explicit the distinction between the 'determinants of health' and the 'determinants of health inequalities'. She makes explicit three distinct meanings of health inequalities in relation to policy action:

- improving the health of poor people
- narrowing the health gaps between the rich and the poor by raising the health of the poor faster
- reducing health gradients so that standards of health enjoyed by the best should be attainable by all

Activity 5.3

1 Are all inequalities in health unfair? What are the major factors to take into account when deciding whether they are inevitable or amenable to change?
2 Describe the differences between the 'determinants of health' and the 'determinants of health inequalities'. What is the implication for policy to support effective action to reduce health inequalities?

Feedback

I No, some inequalities in health are inevitable, such as those caused by genetic or biological factors. The main thing that needs to be taken into account is whether the cause is amenable to an existing, available intervention.

2 Determinants of health are those factors that influence health. In contrast, determinants of health inequalities refers to the distribution of the determinants of health in the population. So, while smoking is a determinant of whether or not someone develops lung cancer, the factors that influence whether or not someone smokes are 'determinants of health inequalities'. The implication is that policies need to address not only the factors that cause ill health but also the factors that cause different sub-groups of the population to be exposed to different levels of risk. One challenge is that policies to reduce the population risk (e.g. smoking cessation activities) may operate differentially and lead to greater health inequalities, even though the overall health of the population has improved.

Explanations for health inequalities

Although research has been conducted into several of the social factors that are known to be associated with health status (e.g. sex, age, ethnicity), the one that has received the greatest attention is socio-economic status.

Four explanations have been proposed for inequalities in health between some socio-economic groups:

- artefact explanations
- natural or social selection
- materialist or structuralist explanations
- cultural/behavioural explanations

Artefact explanations

These suggest that both health and socio-economic status are artificial variables, which have arisen as part of an attempt to measure social phenomena and that the relationship between them may be an artefact and have no causal significance. Such explanations point out that over time there are fewer people in the poorest social classes and therefore this accounts for the persistence of health inequalities. Because of poor data, it is hard to determine whether there is a relationship between social class and health over time. More recent research has shown that other indicators of disadvantage, such as housing tenure, level of education and income, all show a similar pattern of health inequalities, which would suggest that inequalities in health are not an artefact. Nonetheless, measuring social class accurately is important both in terms of being able to monitor the existence of health inequalities and to find ways of reducing them. While statistical artefacts may well contribute to the persistence of health inequality measures, few people accept they can explain all the differences.

Natural or social selection

In this theory, class is considered the dependent (rather than the independent) variable and health is given more causal significance. Thus, class acts as a filter of people and sorts them according to many assets, one of which is health. In other words, the healthiest people are in the most affluent class and therefore have the lowest mortality. It is also postulated that people who have diseases 'sink' to the lower social classes and those who overcome disease move up the social classes. The main argument against this explanation is that there is not enough social mobility (movement of people between classes) to explain much of the difference in health status.

Materialist or structuralist explanations

Such explanations refer to the link between exploitation, poor education and poverty associated with the most deprived classes. In other words, the distribution of health mirrors the distribution of resources. Poverty is taken as a relative concept. There are still many people who are unable to attain the standard of living that the majority of the population shares. This group may also be relatively disadvantaged in relation to the risks of illness or accident, or the factors that promote health. For example, communication about healthy diets may not be in an appropriate style of language for this group. Materialist or structuralist explanations suggest that although levels of health are improving for people in the lower classes, by the time they have caught up to a particular level, the higher social classes have moved further ahead.

Cultural/behavioural explanations

This approach is based on the idea that it is an individual's lifestyle that leads to poor health status. Lifestyles include, for example, whether people smoke, how much they drink, whether they have a poor diet and whether they take exercise. The explanation focuses on the individual and their personal characteristics – intelligence, skills, physical and mental qualities. Some people see behaviour that is conducive to good or bad health as being an intrinsic part of social structures or styles of life. This explanation is seen by some as 'victim blaming', in that people are seen as being responsible for factors which disadvantage them but over which they often have no control.

 Activity 5.4

Considering these four explanations for the existence of inequalities, what might be the role of health promotion in tackling health inequalities?

Feedback

There will never be one answer to tackling health inequalities. Successful strategies will be those which have fully assessed the range and nature of inequalities that exist and apply a range of solutions to fit the context. Health promotion strategies therefore need to be multi-faceted and usually long term.

Central government departments need socio-economic classifications systems because they provide convenient summaries of complex data relevant to the analysis of health inequalities and thus to policy formulation, targeting and evaluation.

Summary

You have learnt about the variety of influences on health, from physiological and biological processes at one end, through lifestyle and environment to political and social structures at the other. Differences in health status among groups in society give rise to inequalities in health. These inequalities can be explained in four ways. There is an ongoing debate about the relative importance of these explanations.

References

Barker DJP (1998) *Mothers, Babies and Disease in Later Life*, 2nd edn. Edinburgh: Churchill Livingstone

Bartley M, Power C, Blane D, Davey Smith G, Shipley M (1994) Birth weight and later socio-economic disadvantage: evidence from the 1958 British cohort study, *British Medical Journal* 309: 1475–8

Dahlgren G, Whitehead M (1991) Policies and strategies to promote social equity in health (mimeo). Stockholm: Institute for Future Studies.

Department of Health (2003) *Tackling Health Inequalities: A Programme for Action*. London: Department of Health

Graham H (2001) The Health Variations programme and the public health agenda. *Health Variations: The Official Newsletter of the ESRC Health Variations Programme*, Issue Seven, April. Lancaster: Lancaster University

Graham H (2004) Social determinants and their unequal distribution: clarifying policy understandings, *The Millbank Quarterly* 82(1): 101–2004

Harris E, Sainsbury P, Nutbeam D (eds.) (1999) *Perspectives on Health Inequity*. Sydney, NSW: Australian Centre for Health Promotion

Lalonde M (1974) *A New Perspective on the Health of Canadians: A Working Document*. Ottawa: Government of Canada

Marmot MG, Rose G, Shipley M, Hamilton PJS (1978) Employment grade and coronary heart disease in British civil servants, *Journal of Epidemiology and Community Health* 32: 244–9

McGinnis JM, Williams-Ruso P, Knickman JR (2002) The case for more active policy attention to health promotion. *Health Affairs* 21(2) (available at: http://content.healthaffairs.org/cgi/reprint/21/2/78)

Townsend P, Davidson N, Whitehead M (1988) *Inequalities in Health* (The Black Report and the Health Divide). London: Pelican

World Health Organization (1998) *Health21: Health for All in the 21st Century*. Copenhagen: WHO Regional Office for Europe

World Health Organization (2003) *The Solid Facts: Social Determinants of Health*. Copenhagen: WHO (available at: http://www.who.dk/document/e81384.pdf)

Further reading

Further detail on the differences between health inequalities and health equity can be found at: http://ftp.who.dk/Document/PAE/conceptsrpd414.pdf

Further details of the issues relating to the definitions of health inequalities can be found in Graham and Kelly (2004) at: http://www.publichealth.nice.org.uk/documents/health_inequalities_concepts.pdf

6 Political and ethical considerations

Overview

You have already learnt that health promotion raises political and ethical issues which need to be taken into account for health promotion to be effective and accepted. These include issues linked to the relationship between individuals and society, who has the right to decide, and the basis on which health promotion is justified. Taking these as a starting point, you will look at some theoretical approaches for considering such issues in political and ethical philosophy, and how they are resolved in practice.

Learning objectives

After working through this chapter, you will be able to:

- **describe some key political and ethical issues relevant to health promotion**
- **be able to relate these issues to some alternative philosophical approaches and consider their usefulness in resolving these health promotion questions**
- **consider how these political and ethical questions are resolved in practice**

Key terms

Beneficence Doing good; active kindness.

Liberalism The rights of the individual should be respected to enable society on a whole to benefit from the full potential of all its citizens.

Non-maleficence A principle based on avoiding the causation of harm.

Plato's republic Governance by those best qualified to do so.

Utilitarianism A theory of the good (whatever yields the greatest utility or value) and a theory of the right (the right act is that which yields the greatest net utility).

Introduction

There is much scope for political debate and dispute on the ends and means of health promotion, and this is something that health professionals need to be aware of in their work. First, over the result to be attained – what is good health? This may seem like a straightforward question but, as you have seen in Chapter 1, in practice people may have different understandings of what health means in practice. Examples could include those linked to self-image (such as obesity and nutrition), behavioural choices (such as smoking, alcohol or drug taking), sexual behaviour (linked to sexually transmitted diseases), or mental health (and attitudes towards depression or suicide). And where there are differences, this leads to questions about whose definition of health should take precedence. The health professional? The individual concerned? Society as a whole?

Second, there may also be differences over the means used for promoting or achieving health. Political questions will arise in particular for those cases where the health-related behaviour of one person has an impact on the health of another. For example, smoking, alcohol (linked to violence) and vaccination (where the benefit is also for the surrounding population). There is also the issue of the cost of treating avoidable ill health and how far the solidarity of the wider community gives people a right to impose their views on the individuals depending on that solidarity.

Third, health is affected by factors such as unemployment, housing, access to essential services, education and the environment. Action to improve health will require political decisions in these areas and the balancing of different priorities against each other. For example, there may be economic or commercial costs to action to promote health.

Looking at these areas of potential conflict, it is clear that there must be some mechanism for resolving differences of view as with other choices about the organization of society as a whole and the limits on the behaviour of individuals within it. This brings you to the political philosophy and organization of the society in which you live and work, as these political mechanisms and values will be what determines the outcomes of these different values in practice. Questions related to health and behaviour are among the most sensitive questions of modern political life and thus it is essential for health professionals to be aware of the wider context to their work.

 Activity 6.1

1 Identify some political and ethical issues related to your area of work or study in health promotion. How are these issues resolved in practice?
2 What political or ethical frameworks are used by you or by others in your area of work or study? Are they compatible?

 Feedback

1 There are likely to be quite a wide range of potential issues, including those described. However, their political or ethical dimension may not be immediately obvious; they may not necessarily be considered through formal political or ethical structures but may be presented in a wide variety of different ways, depending on their specific context. How issues are presented will also affect how they are resolved in practice. People may also present issues in different ways (for example, as a matter of

individual choice rather than as a health issue) depending on the outcome that they would prefer.

2 Many different political and ethical frameworks are mentioned in everyday life. These are not limited to explicit political ideologies. Economic systems (socialism, capitalism) may also be linked to certain political values. Different societies may have established values on certain issues. One clear example is religion; different religious beliefs involve different ethical approaches and may also have an impact on what mechanisms the people concerned accept for resolving conflicts.

A perfect society?

Questions about resolving different values and priorities within society are fundamental and have, therefore, been considered from the earliest works of political philosophy. For the first approach to addressing these issues, you can go back to one of the earliest works of political philosophy – Plato's *The Republic*, written over 3000 years ago in Greece. This was a time of city-states, where different cities within the relatively small geographical area around the Aegean organized themselves quite differently, with consequently much discussion about what the best means of organization was. *The Republic* sets out Plato's answer, a perfect society – the Republic – which is governed by those best qualified to do so: the Guardians.

Plato's argument is that where some activity can be done better by people with more expertise, the best approach is to choose someone who has the appropriate expertise, put them in charge and do as they say. Therefore, the best way to ensure that society is run as well as possible is to select the most capable people, give them all appropriate training and put them in charge; these people are the Guardians, and they direct the behaviour of everyone else.

This is the ultimate vision of society in which decisions are taken based on expertise and evidence. Government is seen as an activity based on knowledge which can be done well or badly, like any other profession. Plato therefore argues that you should logically prefer it to be done well, and thus give the power of decision making to those best qualified to exercise it; you should have the same type of relationship to the Guardians as patients have with their doctor.

Giving power to a small minority on the basis of some expertise or ability does not leave much room for democracy. This is entirely intentional by Plato, who did not view democratic rule as a good thing but rather as encouraging factionalism and selfishness. This 'perfect society' may seem quite alien, with its disregard for individual freedoms and exclusion of most members of society from its governance. Nevertheless, though the society that Plato describes is very different from modern societies, the questions he raises are still relevant today.

Particularly relevant for health promotion is the tension between taking decisions on the basis of expertise or taking decisions on the basis of the majority view of all citizens, regardless of their knowledge or expertise in the area. In Plato's time, there were major advances towards a more scientific and empirical understanding of the world. This was part of the context in which Plato considered that good government should be based on expertise, not just the majority view. Similarly today, we increasingly seek scientifically based explanations and remedies for the problems that confront us, and place great trust in those who have the expertise to analyse and recommend on a scientific basis. The power of the Guardians of Plato's Republic prompted the question 'who will guard the Guardians?', and the same question applies to the authority of health professionals and other experts today. After all, if expertise is the basis of authority, this leads to questions about the basis of this expertise – how we know what the correct analysis or action is.

 Activity 6.2

1 What are the advantages and disadvantages of giving power to experts to decide? Give examples of areas outside health promotion of each approach.
2 How can the authority or expertise of experts be monitored or judged?

 Feedback

1 Advantages of giving power to experts to decide are mostly focused around the *outcome*; someone with expert knowledge of a technical area should produce a better outcome than decisions made without that expertise, all other things being equal. However, there are limits to where this will be the case, which your examples of disadvantages should reflect. In particular, expertise is only useful where the issue for decision is one where technical knowledge is *relevant* – not the case for a conflict of values, for example. And the technical knowledge of the area should be *sufficient* to give a clear answer; where there is disagreement between experts or knowledge is limited, other approaches are required.

Also, decisions by experts may not be appropriate where the process of deciding is itself important – for example, where commitment is required from other people for the decision to be implemented. If people have not been able to choose for themselves or at least been part of a decision-making process which they perceive as fair, they will be less likely to feel committed to implementing a decision in practice. For example, most modern societies take democratic approval as being the ultimate political endorsement for decisions, not expert views; your counter-examples to government by experts could be any area of decision by majority vote. However, there are some areas where decisions are left to experts; having interest rates set by an independent central bank would be one example.

2 On monitoring the authority or expertise of experts, your answer might consider mechanisms such as making the basis for expert decisions open, so that others with expertise can also analyse them; and perhaps mechanisms whereby experts regulate themselves. You may also consider what standards are required of experts, and how these can be upheld – through examples such as professional associations of health professionals or other professions, perhaps.

Utilitarianism or consequence-based theory

Utilitarianism is a suggested theoretical framework for morality, law and politics which accepts the principle of utility as the only basis of ethics. Utilitarianism is both a theory of the good and a theory of the right. As a theory of the good, utilitarianism is welfarist – that is, the good is whatever yields the greatest utility (pleasure, satisfaction, or in reference to an objective list of values). As a theory of the right, utilitarianism is consequentialist – that is, the right act is that which yields the greatest net utility. The origins of this theory can be found in the writings of Jeremy Bentham and John Stuart Mill.

Utilitarians offer many examples from daily life to show that we all engage in a utilitarian method of calculating what should be done by balancing goals and resources and considering the needs of everyone affected. Utilitarians claim that their theory 'renders explicit and systematic what is already implicit in everyday deliberation and justification' (Beauchamp and Childress, 1994).

The principle of utility is the ultimate standard for all utilitarians, although recently there has been argument as to whether this pertains to particular acts, in particular circumstances, or to general rules that determine which actions are right and which are wrong. *Rule* utilitarians consider the consequences of adopting rules, whereas *Act* utilitarians disregard rules and justify their acts by appealing directly to the principle of utility. For the rule utilitarian, an act's conformity to a justified rule makes it right and the rule is in no case expendable, even when following it in that particular situation does not maximize utility. For the act utilitarian, moral rules may be useful as rough guidelines but are expendable if they do not promote utility.

Worthington Hooker was a prominent nineteenth-century doctor and rule utilitarian. He addressed the rule of telling the truth as follows:

The good which may be done by deception in a few cases, is almost as nothing compared with the evil which it does in many, when the prospect of its doing good was just as promising as it was in those in which it succeeded. And when we add to this the evil which would result from a general adoption of a system of deception, the importance of strict adherence to the truth in our intercourse with the sick, even on the ground of expediency, becomes incalculably great.

(cited in Beauchamp and Childress, 1994)

Richard Lamm, a former governor of Colorado, gives a good example of the act utilitarian's point of view (Beauchamp and Childress, 1994). He observed that in view of the increasing financial costs of health care, the terminally ill have 'a duty to die and get out of the way with all of our machines and artificial hearts and everything else'. Naturally, this apparent disregard for the moral rules which protect the public's rights provoked a public outcry, but 'in context, he was giving an act utilitarian answer to what he correctly referred to as an ethical question'. Act utilitarians consider many of the moral questions raised by technological developments impossible to address in terms of traditional moral rules and it has many strengths, hence its popularity among ethicists working in health policy and practice. The requirement for objective assessment of the interests of all concerned and of impartial choice to maximize good outcomes for these are apparently desirable norms of policy making. Utilitarianism is also beneficence-based, seeing morality in terms of promoting welfare. Utilitarianism may appear to demand more than the rules of common morality, but this apparent weakness is also described by Beauchamp and Childress (1994) as a 'hidden strength': 'In many circumstances the utilitarian makes a compelling case in advising us to rely less on everyday convictions and more on judgments of overall benefit'.

Liberalism and individual freedom

An alternative approach to resolving values and priorities in society is to focus not on the overall ideal outcome to be attained, as with Plato, but on the rights of the individual. This 'liberal' approach of individual rights and the balance between the individual and society at large was articulated in particular by John Stuart Mill (1806–1873), and set out at the start of his essay *On Liberty*:

The object of this Essay is to assert one very simple principle, as entitled to govern absolutely the dealings of society with the individual in the way of compulsion and control, whether the means used be physical force in the form of legal penalties or the moral coercion of public opinion. That principle is, that the sole end for which mankind are warranted, individually or collectively, in interfering with the liberty of action of any of their number, is self-protection. That the only purpose for which power can be rightfully exercised over any member of a civilised community, against his will, is to prevent harm to others. His own good, either physical or moral, is not a sufficient warrant. He cannot rightfully be compelled to do or forbear because it will make him happier, because, in the opinions of others, to do so would be wise, or even right. There are good reasons for remonstrating with him, or reasoning with him, or persuading him, or entreating him, but not for compelling him, or visiting him with any evil, in case he do otherwise. To justify that, the conduct from which it is desired to deter him must be calculated to produce evil to some one else. The only part of the conduct of any one, for which is amenable to society, is that which concerns others. In the part which merely concerns himself, his independence is, of right, absolute. Over himself, over his own body and mind, the individual is sovereign.

Mill argued that we should respect these freedoms of the individual both to enable him to realize his own potential and to enable society as a whole to benefit from the full potential of all its citizens. Mill only considers that this applies to adults 'in the maturity of their faculties'. For children, Mill considered that society has a specific responsibility to ensure proper education, to enable them to act rationally as adults and, if it fails, then society must bear the consequences. This liberal tradition was articulated alongside the revolutionary developments in industrialization and urbanization in Western Europe. As well as changes in economic structure, these times also brought major change in social organization, with greater individual freedom both economically and politically, and erosion of the established mechanisms for social control and standards. The liberal tradition gave a philosophical expression to these changes, and still forms a large part of the modern political framework of Western societies.

This philosophical approach sets a clear limit to the role of society in attempting to shape the behaviour of the individual – a limit which is particularly applicable to health issues. Expertise or knowledge of the consequences of a particular kind of behaviour is no justification for interfering in a person's choices, on this basis. For example, the abuse of alcohol was one of the specific cases cited by Mill as something which might not be ideal behaviour but where society should not intervene unless it led to specific harm to someone else:

No person ought to be punished simply for being drunk; but a soldier or a policeman should be punished for being drunk on duty. Whenever, in short, there is a definite damage, or a definite risk of damage, either to an individual or to the public, the case is taken out of the province of liberty, and is placed in that of morality or law.

Yet this also provides an example of the kind of argument that can be made against this liberal position. One might argue that in practical terms, for people living together in a society the distinction between behaviour which causes harm to others and behaviour which is purely private is not as clear as Mill suggests – or at least, that the boundary of what does not affect others needs to be drawn much more narrowly than Mill describes. To continue the example of alcohol misuse, when someone drinks too much and causes harm to themselves, they also cause a burden on society through the efforts of those called on to treat them and the cost of providing health care for them. Does this mean that they are in fact causing harm to others and therefore that social direction of their behaviour is justified?

For Mill, the answer seems to be clearly 'no':

But with regard to the merely contingent, or, as it may be called, constructive injury which a person causes to society, by conduct which neither violates any specific duty to the public, nor occasions any perceptible hurt to any assignable individual except himself; the inconvenience is one which society can afford to bear, for the sake of the greater good of human freedom.

But this position is contested, with proponents of stronger social intervention on issues such as tobacco and alcohol arguing that the overall cost of these behaviours for society justifies interference with individual liberties in this area. This is another area where different values come into conflict when considering specific issues of the politics and ethics of health promotion.

 Activity 6.3

1 What are the advantages and disadvantages of liberalism and only intervening where necessary to prevent harm to others? Consider how some specific health promotion issues would be addressed on this basis.
2 Mill argues that these freedoms only apply to adults 'in the maturity of their faculties' – how should others be treated?

 Feedback

1 Advantages of this approach include *clarity*; this provides a clear test for when intervention is justified. It also respects the rights of the individual and avoids many of the disadvantages of decisions by experts as described above.

Disadvantages are that this has quite significant *limits for health promotion*, which frequently focuses on the good of the individual themselves, which is precisely where Mill argues intervention is not justified. Moreover, even in cases where some action causes harm to others but without intent and without harming a specific individual (which might be the case for environmental damage, for example), Mill seems to argue that intervention is not justified.

However, one important issue to note is that of *consent*. Following this approach does not mean that health promotion aimed at the good of the individual cannot be undertaken, only that it cannot be imposed without their agreement. As set out in the first extract from *On Liberty*, Mill agrees that seeking the agreement of the individual is reasonable; what Mill argues against is compelling someone against their will for their own good. Thus the main limit on health promotion under this approach comes from actions involving some element of obligation – in particular, laws, regulations or other exercise of official authority.

2 This is also relevant for *children* and others who are not capable of making their own decisions, for whatever reason; the key issue is that these people are not able to decide for themselves what is in their own interest and thus there is a greater responsibility on others to make those decisions for them. You should consider who should make those decisions (such as parents or guardians for children) and why. Mill also raises the issue of education and preparing children for life as adults and making their own choices; your answer should address what kind of education would be proper preparation from a health promotion perspective.

The four principles approach

Beauchamp and Childress (1994) defend what is termed the *four principles approach* to health care ethics (also known by its opponents as *principalism*). The principles they describe derive from 'considered judgements' in the common morality and medical traditions. The four clusters of principles are:

1 *Respect for autonomy*: this requires respecting the decision-making capacities of autonomous persons. Many philosophers agree that morality presupposes autonomous actors but emphasizes different themes associated with this autonomy. Beauchamp and Childress (1994) describe the autonomous individual as acting freely 'in accordance with a self-chosen plan, analogous to the way an independent government manages its territories and sets its policies'. On the other hand, 'a person of diminished autonomy . . . is in at least some respect controlled by others or incapable of deliberating or acting on the basis of his or her desires and plans'. Almost all theories of autonomy consider two conditions essential to this: liberty and agency. Nonetheless, they do not necessarily agree as to the meaning of these two conditions.

2 *Non-maleficence*: avoiding the causation of harm. It is closely associated in medical ethics with the maxim *Primum non nocere*: 'Above all, do no harm'. In health care, a decision-making framework for situations which may involve life-sustaining procedures and assistance in dying, for example, is necessary. Beauchamp and Childress (1994) defend a framework centred on 'an interpretation of the principle of non-maleficence that sanctions, rather than suppresses quality of life judgments', allowing public and professionals, under certain conditions, to accept or decline treatment having weighed the advantages and disadvantages of this.

3 *Beneficence*: providing benefits and measuring benefits against risks and costs. 'No sharp breaks exist on the continuum from the non-infliction of harm to the provision of benefit, but principles of beneficence potentially demand more . . . because agents must take positive steps to help others, not merely refrain from harmful acts'. Beauchamp and Childress (1994) describe two principles of beneficence: positive beneficence, which 'requires the provision of benefits', and utility, which requires that 'benefits and drawbacks be balanced'. (The principles of non-maleficence and beneficence are sometimes treated as a single principle.)

4 *Justice*: distributing benefits, risks and costs fairly. Inequalities in access to health care are frequently raised as a moral problem in debates on social justice. In addressing this issue, it is difficult to 'balance and reconcile goals such as the freedom to choose a health plan, equal access to health care, health promotion, a free-market economy, social efficiency, and the beneficent state'. Someone who has a just claim 'has a right, and therefore is due something'. Addressing an injustice involves righting a wrongful act or omission that 'denies people benefits to which they have a right or fails to distribute burdens properly'. All theories of justice demand that equals must be treated equally and unequals must be treated unequally. For this reason, the principle of justice is sometimes called the principle of formal equality.

In addition, Beauchamp and Childress (1994) describe rules which specify principles and serve as a guide to action. The first of these is *substantive rules* of telling the truth – confidentiality, privacy, the fair allocation and rationing of health care, and so on. An example of a rule that specifies the principle of respect for autonomy would be, 'Follow the patient's advance directive whenever it is clear and relevant'. The second type of rule is *authority rules*. Rules of *surrogate authority* determine who should make decisions for incompetent persons and those of *professional authority* decide who should assume responsibility for overriding or accepting patients' decisions in cases where these are potentially damaging. Finally, rules of *distributional authority* determine who should make decisions about the distribution of resources. The third type of rule is *procedural rules*, which establish procedures to be followed when, for example, determining eligibility for medical resources or reporting grievances to higher authorities.

Universal principles of justice?

Given these different possible approaches, is there a way of agreeing on a single common philosophical approach for philosophical principles underlying the relationship between individuals and wider society? One modern proposal was through the work of John Rawls. He attempted to describe a process through which general rational principles for organizing society could be developed.

The starting point is to imagine ourselves outside society (behind what Rawls describes as the 'veil of ignorance'), developing principles by which society should be organized – *without* knowing what position we will ourselves have in that society, or what our abilities will be. The idea of this is to develop principles which we would accept as being universally just, and reasonable for all members of society.

On this basis, Rawls (1971) argues for the following principles:

- each individual is to have a right to the greatest equal liberty compatible with a like liberty for all
- social and economic inequalities are to be attached to offices and positions open to all under conditions of fair equality of opportunity; and such inequalities are justified only if they benefit the worst off

From a health promotion perspective, the first of these principles is the most relevant. As with Mill and the liberal approach, this emphasizes the freedom of the individual. However, this principle contains an important counter-balance – the requirement that all individuals can have the same freedom. If the freedom concerned is not also open to others, then it cannot be open to any. But if it is possible for everyone to have the same degree of liberty, then they should.

By being based purely on a rational analysis detached from individual interest, this theory aims to present a set of common principles which could provide a reference point in considering conflicts and difficult issues, without depending on the particular preferences of the individuals concerned. This seems to be a set of principles that are sufficiently general that they could be widely accepted. By being based purely on a rational analysis, these should in principle share a basis to which everyone could agree. However, that may be part of their problem. A difficulty with very broad principles such as these is that by being sufficiently general to be accepted, they also become so general that they no longer provide a clear guide to resolving specific issues. The first principle of each individual having the greatest equal liberty compatible with a like liberty for all is one which could produce quite different outcomes. Different people are willing to accept different levels of risk and thus would consider different levels of liberty as being reasonable.

 Activity 6.4

What might the principle of 'each individual having a right to the greatest equal liberty compatible with a like liberty for all' mean in practice in the context of health promotion? You may like to consider examples of the misuse of drugs or alcohol.

 Feedback

Your answer is likely to show that this principle could be used to justify quite different approaches. Key factors determining different perceptions of reasonable liberty would include levels of risk that are considered acceptable (some people will be quite willing to accept moderate levels of risk rather than have their liberties curtailed, whereas others would prefer risks to be reduced to a minimum as far as possible), and the linked issue of how they perceive relative values over time – how they compare a small impact now with a larger impact in the future (such as the pleasure of smoking now compared with the potential impact of cancer in the future).

Resolving political and ethical considerations in practice

As you will have seen, there are a wide range of possible approaches to considering political and ethical considerations. You have learnt about several, each of which is reflected to some extent in modern political discussion, and with their advantages and disadvantages.

Each of these approaches is reflected to a certain extent in modern political discussion, without any of them being universally agreed, and with many other possible approaches also being widespread. Different approaches include different religious beliefs, which can be particularly relevant for those whose work has a 'scientific' basis (such as health care expertise), as this can lead to quite different perceptions of issues.

This is not just a matter of philosophical discussion, however. It becomes an important question for health promotion, especially when carried out with or on behalf of public authorities or in pursuit of a public good. Health promotion by or on behalf of public authorities can involve some element of compulsion and even when it does not, it is often perceived as having a coercive element. It is thus important to have not just the agreement of individuals but also, where relevant, the agreement of society as a whole. Of course, there will be a general framework for political and ethical values expressed in the legal framework of the country concerned, which can be taken as describing the accepted rules for that environment. However, this is unlikely to address all the issues that can arise in health promotion. For example, the health impact of particular measures may be unclear or disputed. And even when the scientific evidence about the health consequences of a particular action are clear, individuals may still prefer to make choices which conflict with that advice. Health-related decisions may also conflict with other values (such as moral values) or other interests, requiring some means for making decisions.

To illustrate these issues, consider the following examples of political and ethical discussion over current issues in health promotion.

Measles, mumps and rubella (MMR) vaccination

Controversy arose over this vaccine after a link with inflammatory bowel disease and autism was suggested in 1998. Despite broad scientific consensus that there is no evidence of a link between MMR and these conditions, public confidence in the safety of the vaccine was severely undermined and, in the UK, uptake declined by 8 per cent from the peak coverage of 92 per cent in 1995. The British government decided not to provide vaccination for each of these conditions individually, citing increased danger both to the children concerned and to others through increased risk of transmission of these diseases, despite the concern of many parents over vaccination for their children with MMR.

Ban on smoking in public places

Several high-income countries have some form of ban on smoking in the workplace or public places, including Ireland, Norway, Malta and some US states, citing the need to protect people (in particular workers) from the harmful effects of second-hand tobacco smoke. Proposals for such bans are often controversial and have been argued against on the grounds of the right of individuals to choose to smoke and the potential harm to commercial establishments from a fall in revenue due to smokers choosing to stay away. There have also been disputes between experts over how much harm second-hand tobacco smoke actually does, although the balance of opinion appears to suggest that there is significant harm.

Measures to reduce the harm from HIV/AIDS

Despite the threat from HIV/AIDS, efforts to reduce HIV transmission frequently encounter conflicts with other values, such as ethical judgements about behaviour with a particular risk of HIV infection, linked moral judgements about some of the groups at particular risk (such as homosexuals or intravenous drug users), or stigmatization of HIV-positive people. Therapies for HIV/AIDS are often relatively costly and have to compete with other priorities for expenditure (in the health area or elsewhere), and with commercial returns for their manufacturers (in the case of pharmaceutical products, for example) and intellectual property and patent protection.

Activity 6.5

  1 What political and ethical issues do these examples raise?
  2 How could they best be resolved?

Feedback

1 These examples all raise many of the issues already discussed in this chapter, such as the tension between expertise and individual choice, and between individual choices and the values of the community.

2 On the issue of MMR vaccination, your answer should identify issues around justifying action on scientific expertise and how to decide between expert judgements on the one hand and the wishes of individuals on the other when they conflict. This also raises issues about individual consent, as a government's decision not to offer the three separate vaccines can be considered to be, in effect, a form of official pressure, as well as the potential for harm to others through diseases transmitted due to lack of vaccination using MMR. You may also refer back to your answer under Activity 6.3 on how society should handle the health choices of children, as these vaccines are given at a young age and thus decisions are being made by parents or guardians.

On the issue of banning smoking in public places, this raises issues about the balance between individual consent and possible harm to others – also in terms of health, or sometimes in terms of other factors (such as the economic harm to commercial establishments). This is also a clear example of using political processes (legislation) to achieve a health promotion goal, including use of the coercive power of the state. You may have considered whether it is possible to compare different interests when they are of different types (such as by putting a monetary value on non-monetary interests to enable comparisons). This issue also again raises questions about how to decide between different expert viewpoints, given the different views of experts over the harm from second-hand tobacco smoke.

On the issue of measures to reduce the harm from HIV/AIDS, this raises issues about conflicting ethical values in particular, and how to resolve them. One particular issue you might consider is where different values are linked to different perceptions of the world and accepted mechanisms for resolving conflicts – such as the tension between scientific and religious explanations, for example, or between formal political structures and other more traditional forms of authority and decision making. Likewise, where resources are limited, mechanisms for deciding between competing priorities are required, both between health priorities and with regard to others.

Summary

You have learnt about political and ethical aspects of health promotion, starting with identifying some of the political and ethical issues that health promotion may raise. You then learnt about five different approaches to considering political issues and the balances to be struck: a perfect society, described by Plato; utilitarianism; liberalism and individual freedom; the four principles approach; and universal principles of justice based on rationality. All of these approaches have advantages and disadvantages and the framework in which health promotion is carried out will involve elements of these and other approaches.

References

Beauchamp TL, Childress JF (1994) *Principles of Biomedical Ethics*, 4th edn. Oxford: Oxford University Press
Mill JS (1986) On Liberty, in Stewart RM, *Readings in Social and Political Philosophy*. Oxford: Oxford University Press
Rawls J (1971) A theory of justice. Cambridge MA: Belknap Press

Further reading

Berger F (1984) *Happiness, Justice, and Freedom: The Moral and Political Philosophy of John Stuart Mill*. Berkeley, CA: University of California Press
Burns JH, Hart HLA (eds.) (1977) *The Introduction to the Principles of Morals and Legislation*. London: Athline Press.
Cribb A, Duncan P (2002) *Health Promotion and Professional Ethics*. Oxford: Blackwell.
Dinwiddy J (1989) *Bentham*. Oxford: Oxford University Press
Elster J (1989) *Nuts and Bolts for the Social Sciences*. Cambridge: Cambridge University Press
Norman R (1998) *The Moral Philosophers: An Introduction to Ethics*, 2nd edn. Oxford: Oxford University Press
Pettit P (1991) Consequentialism, in Singer P (ed.) *A Companion to Ethics*. Oxford: Blackwell
Sabine G (1951) *A History of Political Theory*, 3rd edn. London: George G Harrap and Co
Seedhouse D (1998) *Ethics: The Heart of Health Care*, 2nd edn. Chichester: Wiley

7 Targets, standards and indicators

Overview

In this chapter, you will consider why it is necessary to set targets for health promotion and what the evidence tells you about the most effective ways of doing so. Other concepts covered include: the interplay between targets, indicators and standards in health promotion. Examples of public health targets, indicators and standards and their applications are reviewed. Finally, the implications for national and local action are considered.

Learning objectives

After working through this chapter, you will be better able to:

- **understand key concepts associated with target setting in health promotion**
- **be familiar with the differences between goals, aims, objectives, targets and standards and how they interrelate**
- **appreciate why target setting and the targeting of health promotion interventions is key to the success of programmes**

Key terms

Aim An expanded and refined version of a goal that sets out the means by which the end point, in general terms, is to be attained.

Goal A general statement of intent, usually based on a set of principles or values.

Indicator An attribute or variable used in the measurement of change.

Objective Concrete and specific elaboration of an aim.

Standard The basis for comparison or a reference point against which other things can be evaluated.

Target Similar to an objective in that it usually contains a quantifiable measure set to be achieved by a particular date.

Introduction

Not withstanding the real and persistent health inequalities that exist between and within communities, over the last hundred years the health of the populations of high-income countries have improved dramatically. To a lesser, but significant extent, the same is true for low- and middle-income countries.

What led to this great advance was a host of interventions including improved housing, sanitation, food supply and safety, better working conditions and employment rights, immunization programmes and family planning services. These improvements were often made possible, and at the same time contributed to, the general economic development of communities and countries. The development of welfare provision and health services also made substantial contributions. One of the key factors that drove forward this improvement was the setting of often challenging but achievable targets for improvement. History teaches that the setting of well-informed health targets is one of the key mechanisms for not only raising expectations of better health but also delivering improvements.

The less healthy in many societies, however, are not just lagging behind the better off – they are not catching up, and in many cases, they are falling further behind. Figure 7.1 illustrates the growing mortality gap between social classes in England and Wales between 1930 and 1993. While the growing disparity between social classes is clear, it is also clear that it is possible to reduce such disparity as seen by the narrowing of the gap that took place in the early 1970s.

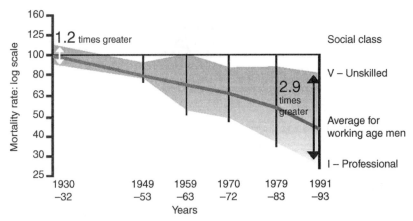

Figure 7.1 The widening mortality gap between the social classes in England and Wales

* 1979–83 excludes 1981. Men of working age varies according to year (either aged 15 or 20 to age 64 or 65)

Source: Office of National Statistics

Many governments and organizations have made poor progress in health improvement for several reasons:

- focusing too much on cure and too little on prevention
- not developing a robust evidence-based approach to health promotion interventions

- emphasizing short-term thinking and project-focused approaches as opposed to long-term strategic planning and programme approaches
- failing to coordinate and make best use of all state and civic assets to tackle health challenges
- failing to identify and share effective practice
- adopting paternalistic attitudes to health issues dominated by professional prescriptions for action

Two additional reasons have been a failure to invest sufficiently in developing health and epidemiological surveillance systems and failing to invest in effective target setting that is integrated as part of a long-term commitment to developing a performance culture focused on continuous progressive improvement. Effective health target setting is one of the key elements of a sophisticated and effective health improvement strategy and is the subject of this chapter.

Establishing a common language for target setting

The setting of health targets, while being a fairly universal feature of health improvement planning, is more an art than a science. There is a fair amount of agreement about the differences, applications and interplay between the terms 'goals', 'aims', 'objectives', 'targets', 'indicators' and 'standards'. The following should act as a guide rather than a set of absolute definitions.

The difference in the meaning and application of these terms may seem unimportant but this is not the case. Clarity in both selecting and applying these terms is vital if there is to be corresponding clarity about what is to be achieved, by when and by whom, and why this is important. In addition, a careful and consistent setting out of health promotion goals, aims, objectives, targets, indicators and standards will help to ensure that an intervention stands the best chance of being implemented successfully and evaluated fairly.

Goal

A goal is a general statement of intent usually based on a set of principles or values. Goals set out what should be achieved. A good example is the United Nations' (2000) Millennium Declaration:

1 eradicate extreme poverty and hunger
2 achieve universal primary education
3 promote gender equality and empower women
4 reduce child mortality
5 improve maternal health
6 combat HIV/AIDS, malaria and other diseases
7 ensure environmental sustainability
8 develop a global partnership for development

Aim

An aim is an expanded and refined version of a goal that sets out the means by which the end point, in general terms, is to be attained (and which is believed to be attainable). An example of a health promotion aim derived from a health goal, such as the fourth Millennium Development Goal, would be: To reduce child mortality by instigating an international programme of infant nutritional supplementation in order to increase calorific intake and reduce malnutrition.

Target

A target usually contains concrete and quantifiable measures that are to be achieved by a particular date. For example, 'to reduce the numbers of smokers from workless households by 25% by 2007'. Targets differ from objectives in that they often carry with them some implied or actual threat of penalty for failure to attain them, or incentive for fully meeting the target. Targets are discussed further in a moment.

Objective

Objectives are concrete and specific elaboration of aims and they must be measurable.

Indicator

Bull and Hamer (2001) define indicators as follows: 'Indicators are selected to measure movement towards or away from a pre-defined target. They are attributes or variables used in the measurement of change, e.g. number of low income women attending smoking cessation clinics'. This definition makes it clear that indicators differ from targets in that they are more concerned with monitoring progress rather than setting out an achievement to be attained.

Standard

A standard is the basis for comparison or a reference point against which other things can be evaluated. Standards set the measure for all subsequent work. Standards are established or widely recognized as a model of authority or excellence, often developed and endorsed by groups of experts. For example, a standard focused on oral health could state that all dental health educators have to be qualified and certificated as being fit to practise before being allowed to work with individuals or community groups unsupervised.

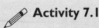 **Activity 7.1**

In what order would the goals, aims, objectives, targets, indicators and standards normally be developed for a health promotion programme?

Feedback

> It would be normal to start with what broadly it is hoped to be achieved – that is, a goal. You would then consider the overall aims, usually only one or two. From this, you would develop a set of objectives that detail in specific terms what is actually going to be done and by when. This means that normally you are working from the broad concepts to the defined actions.
>
> Often what happens is that health promoters respond to targets that have been set by national and local governments, though these may not be in line with local needs and priorities.

The nature of targets

Targets are an important part of any strategic planning. Targets are a way of ensuring that resources and effort are directed at improving health status in an explicit and measurable way. Targets can inspire and motivate, serve as a technical tool for the development of indicators to measuring progress and offer a way of rationalizing and making explicit complex policy decisions.

Target development and setting can also be a vehicle for consensus building among partners about priorities for health improvement. The evidence suggests that targets are helpful to both policy makers and operational staff. Targets help by tracking success or failure and informing the development of new programmes of work. Evidence and experience also show that broad inclusion in the development and collection of information used to monitor progress helps to avoid both data sabotage and measuring the wrong things. In general terms, less is more when it comes to target development and setting. A few key targets are more likely to bring about improved service delivery than a large battery of targets that result in superficial review and progress checking. Targets also need to be SMART:

- Specific
- Measurable
- Achievable
- Relevant
- Time bound

Other key issues about the development of targets include:

- the importance of independent verification of progress towards targets
- the challenge of coordinating progress when responsibility is shared among many partners
- gaming and the manipulation of data
- creating perverse incentives
- the importance of professional judgement in setting, interpreting and developing targets
- the importance of ownership, because without ownership, target fixing and sabotage are possible

The language of risk

There is a need for clarity and consistency in the application of language and its underlying conceptual basis. As Naidoo and Wills (2004) state:

> The concept of targeting rests on a notion of risk. Epidemiologists assess risk in terms of the statistical probability of adverse events or death occurring. The link between this and certain identified factors can be expressed on a continuum from negligible to high. Lay people assess risk in the light of their personal experience and similarly may see actions as high or low risk, although this does not necessarily correspond with epidemiologists' assessment.

The importance of a common language of risk has also been highlighted by Calman (1996), who suggested standardization of terms that quantify risk (Table 7.1).

Table 7.1 Terms describing and quantifying risk

Term used	Risk estimate	Example
High	Greater than 1:100	Mother–child transmission of HIV
Moderate	Between 1:100 and 1:1000	Smoking ten cigarettes per day
Low	Between 1:1000 and 1:10,000	Road accident
Very low	Between 1:10,000 and 1:100,000	Leukaemia
Minimal	Between 1:100,000 and 1:1,000,000	Vaccination-associated polio
Negligible	Over 1:1,000,000	Hit by lightening

Source: Calman (1996)

The link between risk and the targeting of health promotion interventions was described by Geoffrey Rose (1981) as the 'prevention paradox'. If exposure to the cause of a disease is homogeneous within a population, then case/control studies will fail to detect it. For example, if everyone smoked 20 cigarettes a day, such studies would lead us to conclude that lung cancer was a genetic disease. In some ways this would be true, since the distribution of cases would be determined by individual susceptibility. Rose argues that two distinct but complementary strategies are needed to address the determinants of individual cases of disease and the determinants of incidence within populations. These two strategies are known as the 'high-risk approach' and the 'population approach'. The strategy to reduce individual risk is the high-risk approach, which seeks to protect susceptible individuals. The strategy to reduce incidence is the population approach, which seeks to control the causes of disease. The two approaches are not usually in competition. Both strategies have advantages and disadvantages:

The high-risk approach

This strategy aims to identify those at greatest risk and intervene to lower their risk.

Disadvantages

- difficulties and costs of screening
- not radical, as it does not deal with the cause of the problem
- limited potential for population health improvement
- behaviourally inappropriate, as it does not address social norms that frame health behaviour

Advantages

- intervention appropriate to individuals
- subject motivation is usually high
- medical and implementation staff motivation usually high
- can be a cost-effective use of resources
- benefit–risk ratio favourable for engagement on the part of the patient

The population approach

This strategy attempts to lower the mean level of risk in the population and shift the whole distribution of exposure in a favourable direction

Disadvantages

- there is only a small benefit for most individuals (prevention paradox)
- may be poor motivation of most subjects
- may be poor motivation of the medical and other staff leading the intervention
- benefit–risk ratio may be 'worrisome' for some individuals

Advantages

- it seeks to remove the root cause of the problem
- large potential for population improvement
- behaviourally appropriate in that it seeks to shift population norms

The prevention paradox relates to the fact that most people in a population approach may receive little benefit even having changed their behaviour. Rose quotes the Framingham coronary heart disease prevention study which showed that if all men aged up to 55 reduced their cholesterol level by 10 per cent, one in 50 would avoid a heart attack but 49 out of 50 would need to eat differently for 40 years and derive no direct benefit in terms of reduced heart attack risk. The prevention paradox makes it clear that a preventive measure that brings much benefit to populations may offer little to each participating individual, but such interventions are still often the most efficient and cost-effective way of improving population health from society's point of view.

 Activity 7.2

Describe the characteristics of the high-risk approach and the population approach for a topic you are familiar with, noting the advantages and disadvantages of each approach.

 Feedback

A high-risk approach will entail identifying and concentrating efforts on those in the population who are found to be at high risk. For example, those with a high body mass index, high blood pressure, or high blood lipid level. In contrast, the population approach will entail attempting to reduce the risk factors in everybody in the population. The advantages and disadvantages, described above, will apply differently depending on the topic you are considering.

Setting and using health promotion targets: a UK case study

The setting of health promotion targets is used in most countries and is also widely used by international organizations such as the World Health Organization. The following health promotion targets were set by the British government in 2004:

Increase life expectancy at birth by 2010 by

- cutting mortality from **heart disease and stroke** plus a 40% reduction in inequalities between areas
- cutting mortality from **cancer** plus a 6% reduction in inequalities between areas
- cutting mortality from **suicide/undetermined injury**

Reduce health inequalities by 10% by 2010

Tackling the underlying determinants by

- reducing **adult smoking**, especially among manual groups
- halting the year-on-year rise in **childhood obesity**
- reducing the **under-18 conception** rate

(Department of Health, 2004)

These and similar targets can be an important symbol of the need for change and can help foster a learning culture within organizations and communities seeking to bring about health improvement. However, targets can also have the effect of distorting services if they are poorly formulated, non-specific or result in severe penalties on service providers who fail to hit targets.

In the UK, a Parliamentary Committee set out in 2003 in *On Target* a clear statement of what it believes should be achieved through the application of targets. Five aspirational roles for target setting were set out:

1 Clear sense of direction and ambitions
2 Focus on delivering results
3 Basis for what is and is not working well
4 Better accountability
5 Move from a measurement culture to a performance culture

However, these aspirations are not always recognized by providers of services and there is often a lack of integration in building a performance culture, which *On Target* perceives as the ultimate goal. A measurement culture is a potential negative consequence of target setting, in that targets can easily become instruments that distort the way services are provided. It is, however, possible to ameliorate the worst consequences of a measurement culture. Strategies to achieve this include ensuring that fewer outcome targets are set and that there is a wide consultation process used to establish targets in the first place. A move away from a 'hit or miss' approach to target setting and a move towards a 'progress' approach will also help. Regular review of the appropriateness of targets and independent assessment of both progress towards targets and their ongoing utility also help to ensure that health promotion targets are a positive force for health improvement.

The emphasis of standards, as well as targets, appears to demonstrate a constancy of policy response in that a balanced package of focused national targets, locally derived targets and an agreed set of standards will be used to monitor performance and help build a performance culture. However, where there is less knowledge about what works, which is often the case with health promotion interventions, setting clear targets and leaving front line staff free to interpret how best to deliver them may be a more effective strategy. The setting of standards of performance is less important and may restrict the development of the most appropriate local responses in these kinds of areas. The interplay between targets and standards is a complex one. What is essential is that there is clarity about both how standards and targets relate to each other and how they will be used to both stimulate best practice and measure the achievement policy goals.

Successful targets setting and targeting health promotion interventions

Targets can be an important symbol of the need to change and can help foster a learning culture within organizations and communities. Additionally, as argued above, targets can help to ensure that resources are devoted to meeting key policy goals. In addition to target setting, it is also important to target health promotion interventions at specific communities or audiences because society is segmented in terms of its wants, desires and health needs. While the targeting of health promotion interventions is not the main focus of this chapter, such targeting is key if further improvements in health are to be realized. Figure 7.2 demonstrates that there are substantial differences within what could erroneously be thought of as a homogeneous group of women born outside the UK. This implies that both target setting and the targeting of interventions to assist people to take up preventive services or change behaviour need to be considered.

In addition to the need to ensure that health promotion targets are sensitive to the needs of different sub-sections of the population, there is also the need to consider the issue of 'risk conditions' when setting targets. The 'population approach' often focuses on risk factors such as smoking, lack of exercise and poor diets, rather than on what have been called 'risk conditions'. Risk conditions relate to the broader environmental and socio-political factors that affect people's health. Such risk conditions include people's housing, employment, income, access to transport and to health care. Given the growing evidence base on the social determinants of ill health, targets to address inequalities in health need to move beyond the setting of specific disease-based or service-specific outcome targets and begin to set targets that relate to what have been termed 'up-stream' health determinants (Whitehead *et al.*, 1998). However, such a determinants or up-stream focus is still essentially operating in what can be called a negative or deficit model of health, focused on the reduction of disease and suffering rather than being focused on the development of positive health. Rather than a problem focus, it has been argued by Harrison *et al.* (2004) that there is a need to develop health targets and intervention strategies that have a positive focus. They argue that such an approach is a logical response for taking forward health improvement and is supported by growing evidence about what works in the promotion of health.

The literature on target setting identifies several criteria for success. These criteria have been summarized by Bull and Hamer (2001) as follows:

- *Credibility*: Targets must find a balance between being realistic – capable of being achieved within the time scale proposed – and being sufficiently ambitious. Experience shows that setting targets that would have been met in any case or setting targets that are over-ambitious fail to motivate the necessary people. This is not to deny the importance of 'early wins', – that is, making early tangible progress.
- *Relevance*: Targets should relate to an overall strategy. They should also relate to clearly identified health problems that are demonstrably amenable to action.
- *Evidence base*: Sufficient evidence should be available about the effectiveness of interventions used to tackle health problems. Targets should relate to interventions that are based on evidence of what works. This evidence can be drawn from scientific research literature, from evidence of 'good practice', as well as expert and lay opinion. The existence of historical data can add to the weight of evidence about what kind of change can be expected over what period. If, for example, a percentage change is required, it should be based on robust baseline data. High-level evidence of effectiveness about specific interventions to tackle health inequalities is often unavailable and highlights the need for more evaluation.
- *Ownership*: Targets should be meaningful and acceptable to all those who are to be responsible for their delivery. The best way to achieve this is to involve all the key players in setting the targets. This is particularly important in the case of targets that require action across sectors for their successful implementation, which is likely to be the case for any targets that relate to tackling health inequalities. Local communities also have a role in setting broad local health priorities. The process of consensus building is an important but often neglected part of target setting but is as important as the technical dimensions of setting targets.

- *Monitoring and evaluation*: The organizations responsible for achieving the target should be clearly identified and lead responsibility assigned. Lead organizations must be given the authority and responsibility to control and influence action to deliver the target. Continuous review mechanisms should be put in place with adequate resources for collection of data to monitor progress. Thought should be given to incentives and to relating the targets to existing performance management frameworks.

In summary, the evidence base on international experience about setting health promotion targets indicates that when there is a strong knowledge base and consensus about intervention methodology, and a high degree of central specification of interventions (for example, setting explicit delivery standards that focus on a few key priorities). Where there is less knowledge and a lack of consensus about what works, management by objectives is more likely to succeed. In these circumstances, the best way forward is to ensure that the setting is clear and there are too many targets, and then leaving more freedom for intervention leaders to interpret how best to deliver in local communities and settings.

 Activity 7.3

Identify a health promotion strategy in your own country and the targets it has set. Consider the strengths, weaknesses, opportunities and threats posed by these.

 Feedback

1 The strengths that you have identified might include: clarity of focus; credibility; realistic and achievable outcomes; focus on delivery; support of a performance culture; freedom to act locally.

2 The weaknesses you have identified could include: meeting national targets predominates over local need; too many targets; unrealistic expectations.

3 The threats might include: restricts local response, a culture that only values achievement of targets; loss of autonomy.

4 The opportunities might include; the rewards for meeting targets, help to secure resources; focuses efforts from a range of stakeholders.

Implications for national and local action

It is the job of policy makers to question how we should proceed in developing and setting health promotion targets. A key element in the development of strategies at both national and local level is the need for them to be developed both from the bottom up and from the centre, in a coordinated way. The key characteristics of such an integrated approach include listening and the development of joint planning mechanisms. As you learnt earlier, the ownership of strategic goals, targets, intervention mechanisms and review systems is important, as is the need to ensure that there is a coordinated inter-departmental and inter-sectoral approach to developing a consensus about which targets should be selected and how they should be achieved.

There are three further implications for both the development and use of effective targets. First, an investment in professional development to build the skills necessary for the development and use of targets. Second, the need to link targets and performance management systems. And, finally, the establishment of mechanisms for coordinating data use, evaluation and research.

There are several reasons why setting local targets is complex:

- It requires an understanding of social, health and asset models of health.
- Local targets need to complement national, regional and, in some cases, international targets.
- Targets need to be set in relation to health promotion issues that are amenable to intervention, and as the state of the evidence base for many interventions is only slowly developing, this can be problematic.
- There is a need to engage with partners in setting and delivering on targets if all local organizations that can make a contribution to bringing about positive change are to be harnessed.

Summary

You have seen that there is a need to consider going beyond traditional disease and deficit models when developing health promotion targets and also to consider targets that relate to the positive development of health. The importance of assessment of the evidence base about the effectiveness of health promotion interventions is also key (and will be addressed further in Chapter 15). There is also a need for inter-sectoral consistency in target setting and review. Targets are important drivers for effective health promotion practice and appear to work best when they are used as part of a more general strategy to develop a performance culture among those responsible for delivering health promotion. Targets need to be seen in this context if they are to be used as part of a process to move beyond a focus on simplistic assessments of success and failure.

References

Bull J, Hamer L (2001) *Closing the Gap: Setting Local Targets to Reduce Health Inequalities.* London: HDA

Calman KC (1996) Cancer: science and society and the communications of risk, *British Medical Journal* 313: 799–802

Department of Health (2004) *Choosing Health: Making Healthier Choices Easier.* London: HMSO

Harrison D, Ziglio E, Levin L, Kasapi E, Morgan A, Brown C (2004) *Assets for Health and Development: The European Programme (AHDEP). Developing a Conceptual Framework.* Venice: WHO European Office for Investment for Health and Development

House of Commons Public Administration Select Committee (July 2003) *'On Target' Government by Measurement.* London: HMSO

Naidoo J, Wills J (2004) *Practicing Health Promotion Dilemmas and Challenges.* London: Baillière Tindall with Royal College of Nursing

Rose G (1981) Strategy of prevention: lessons from cardiovascular disease, *British Medical Journal* 282: 1847–51

United Nations (2000) *Millennium Declaration*. A/RES/55/2, 18 September. New York: UN

Webb R, Richardson J, Esmail A, Pickles A (2004). Uptake of cervical screening by ethnicity and place-of-birth: a population-based cross-sectional study. J Public Health 26: 293–6

Whitehead M, Scott-Samuel A, Dahlgren G (1998) Setting targets to reduce inequalities in health, *The Lancet* 351.

SECTION 3

Public policy

8 Healthy public policy

Overview

In this chapter, you will look at the development of healthy public policy which pays attention to how health is promoted through the actions of decision makers and communities outside the health care sector. You will also learn about the ongoing debates about the concept of healthy public policy.

Learning objectives

After working through this chapter, you will be better able to:

- **understand the historical origins and modern development of the concept of healthy public policy**
- **describe the potential for advocating, developing and implementing healthy public policy**
- **identify constraints on healthy public policy and approaches to overcoming them**

Key term

Healthy public policy An approach characterized by an explicit concern for health and equity in all areas of policy and an accountability for health impact.

The origins of healthy public policy

Healthy public policy has its origins in the development of the 'new public health' and in the changing concepts and principles of health promotion over the last quarter of a century, which you learnt about in Chapters 1 and 2. As you will recall, understanding of what are the most significant influences on health has shifted with changes in the structure and organization of society and the knowledge of causes of disease.

Activity 8.1

From what you learnt in earlier chapters, suggest the four components of an effective policy to improve the health of the public.

Feedback

The four components of public health policy are:

- environmental measures to reduce risks and protect health
- changes in lifestyles and individual behaviour
- immunization, vaccination and effective treatment of diseases
- political, economic and social measures

 Activity 8.2

Reflect on the current emphasis on these aspects in your own country. You will need to consider the following questions:

- Are resources directed mostly at health care or on making the environment healthier and reducing poverty?
- Is health largely thought of as the responsibility of the individual to choose healthy life-styles and seek treatment when necessary, or is it seen more as a collective good?
- What behavioural and environmental factors are having the most influence on health now?

 Feedback

Your notes will be dependent on health policy and provision where you live, but you should have made some observations about the relative level of investment in personal health care and actions on the determinants of health; whether your current govern-ment policy balances efforts to address individual lifestyle with social and environ-mental action and what the current health priorities are.

You also saw in Chapter 2 how the World Health Organization and some national initiatives have encouraged the development of healthy public policies over the past few decades. Their main objectives have been the promotion of lifestyles con-ducive to health, the prevention of disease, and the provision of rehabilitation and health services. These can be seen in the WHO Targets for Health for All published in 1985. There were thirty-eight targets grouped as follows:

- Targets 1–12: Health for All; covering equity, increasing life expectancy and reducing disease
- Targets 13–17: Lifestyles Conducive to Health for All; including Target 13 'Developing Healthy Public Policies', which you will look at in more detail below.
- Targets 18–25: Producing Healthy Environments; including environment, housing and work-related risks
- Targets 26–31: Providing Appropriate Care; with a focus on primary care and the importance of improving the quality of services
- Targets 32–38: Support for Health Development; covering research, informa-tion, education and training, and health technology assessment

As can be seen from this brief listing, the targets are a holistic approach to health improvement, with actions required in all sectors, and a prediction of a requirement for advanced technologies in terms of evidence, education and quality improvement. Target 13 focused on the need to develop healthy public policies:

By 1990, national policies in all Member States should ensure that legislative, administrative, and economic mechanisms provide broad intersectoral support and resources for the promotion of healthy lifestyles and ensure effective participation at all levels of such policy-making. The attainment of this target could be significantly supported by strategic health planning at cabinet level, to cover broad intersectoral issues that affect lifestyle and health, the periodic assessment of existing policies in their relationship to health, and the establishment of effective machinery for public involvement in policy planning and development.

Developments in the definition and understanding of health promotion, as one of the key vehicles to implement the Health for All 2000 (WHO, 1981) strategy, and healthy public policy were moving hand in hand. This is significant in that it underscores the principles and values of the practice of health promotion embedded in Health for All 2000. The WHO (1984) document on concepts and principles and the Ottawa Charter (WHO, 1986) provide the foundation stones for the approach to healthy public policy. The principles of health promotion were defined by the World Health Organization as:

- involving the population as a whole in the context of their everyday life rather than focusing on people at risk for specific disease
- directed towards action on the determinants of health, requiring cooperation between sectors and government
- combining diverse but complementary approaches, including individual communication and education, legislation, fiscal measures, and organizational and community development
- effective community participation
- involvement of health professionals, particularly in primary health care. Although directing action away from health care, health care professionals were not to be 'let off the hook' in terms of their responsibilities

Critiques and defence of healthy public policy

There has been some debate about the meaning of 'healthy public policy' versus 'health promotion policy' – this really depends on whether the term 'health promotion' is being used as the goal of health improvement (in which case they are synonymous) or as the term for a field of endeavour (in which case health promotion policy is more limited to the practice and delivery of health promotion programmes). Some of the dilemmas inherent in the whole approach to healthy public policy have been presciently stated and it is worth reflecting on the directions that have been taken since in the field of health promotion and whether these dilemmas are still relevant in current practice.

The political and moral dilemmas associated with health promotion, as stated by WHO (1984), included:

- the rise of 'healthism' – the ideology that health is the ultimate goal of all life, not the means to a fulfilled and quality life

- individual responsibility for health and the rise of 'victim blaming' rather than action on social and economic conditions
- increases in social and health inequalities as a result of health promotion initiatives being inaccessible to those very sections of the population most disadvantaged
- the professionalization of health promotion – making it a field of specialization to the exclusion of other professionals and lay people

The extract from Targets for Health For All (WHO, 1985) that follows outlines many of the practical aspects that need to be taken into consideration in the implementation of healthy public policy. It is recognition of these techniques that characterizes the practice of health promotion. Although this is now 20 years old, the themes and issues are still pertinent today in the practice of multi-sectoral (partnership) working, which is the bedrock of healthy public policy.

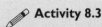 **Activity 8.3**

While reading the extract, make notes as to which issues are still relevant or indeed are still underdeveloped in your country.

 Priorities for the development of policies in health promotion

Health promotion stands for the collective effort to attain health. Governments, through public policy, have a special responsibility to ensure basic conditions for a healthy life and for making the healthier choices the easier choices. At the same time supporters of health promotion within governments need to be aware of the role of spontaneous action for health, i.e. the role of social movements, self-help and self-care, and the need for continuous cooperation with the public on all health promotion issues.

1   *The concept and meaning of 'health promotion'* should be clarified at every level of planning, emphasising a social, economic and ecological, rather than purely physical and mental perspective on health. Policy development in health promotion can then be related and integrated with policy in other sectors such as work, housing, social services and primary health care.

2   *Political commitment to health promotion* can be expressed through the establishment of focal points for health promotion at all levels – local, regional and national. These would be organisational mechanisms for intersectoral co-ordinated planning in health promotion. They should provide leadership and accountability so that, when action is agreed, progress will be secured. Adequate funding and skilled personnel are essential to allow the development of systematic long-term programmes in health promotion.

3   In the development of health promotion policies there must be *continuous consultation, dialogue and exchange of ideas* between individuals and groups, both lay and professional. Policy mechanisms must be established to ensure opportunities for the expression and development of public interest in health.

4 *When selecting priority areas for policy development a review should be made of:*

Indicators of health and their distribution in the population
Current knowledge, skills and health practices of the population
Current policies in government and other sectors

Further an assessment should be made of:

The expected impact on health of different policies and programmes
The economic constraints and benefits
The social and cultural acceptability
The political feasibility of different options

5 *Research support is essential for policy development and evaluation* to provide an under-standing of influences on health and their development, as well as an assessment of the impact of different initiatives in health promotion. There is a need to develop method-ologies for research and analysis, in particular, to devise more appropriate approaches to evaluation. The results of research should be disseminated widely and comparisons made within and between nations.

 Feedback

Your answer will depend on your choice of country. As an example, a response in the UK might be:

- change in the registration requirements for public health specialists to include non-medical people has led the health promotion profession firmly in the direction of specialization
- health inequalities have widened, possibly as a result of the increased uptake of healthy behaviours by the better-off and well educated, a potential negative con-sequence of health promotion
- the need for coordinated planning and integrated policy across sectors is still being understood and there are not enough leaders and skilled personnel
- the characteristics of successful partnership working include attention to communi-cation and dialogue between sectors and with the community
- there is still a need for health impact assessment of policies, cost–benefit analysis of interventions and the development of appropriate evidence of effective interventions in health promotion

---

There is an ongoing debate about some of these issues. Nancy Milio (1986) eloquently dismissed the argument between individual and collective responsi-bility for health as follows: 'Policy is, after all, no more nor less than a collective choice on collective lifestyle that sets the terms for individuals' choices'. That is, politics, democracy and choice about the type of society and lifestyles people wish to lead are all bound together. By being active in decision making and involved in the construction of policy (either directly or through the ballot box), individuals are able to influence these choices. Ron Draper (1987) pointed out that many scep-tics viewed healthy public policy as an idealistic concept, a sort of 'Mom and Apple pie' utopia that just wasn't real. The political challenge necessitated recognizing that:

intersectoral action requires analysis of complex issues and balancing of conflicting interests across a bewildering spectrum of concerns. It is difficult to escape the impression that losers as well as winners will emerge from the introduction of such policies, at least in the short term. Consequently healthy public policy is sometimes dismissed as an impossible dream.

In developing integrated policy through partnerships, several skills are necessary: understanding of the balance of interests at play and high levels of negotiation and communication skills.

The Ottawa Charter (WHO, 1986) reinforced the view that health promoters should concern themselves with policy change, by placing the goal to build public policies which support health at the top of its list of actions to support the implementation of Health for All 2000. And the Adelaide Recommendations (WHO, 1988) consolidated the thinking of how to achieve changes in healthy public policy. In addition to building on the principles and values already outlined, it highlighted four key action areas: supporting the health of women, food and nutrition, tobacco and alcohol, and creating supportive environments. It firmly reinforced the need for intersectoral working and introduced (somewhat tentatively), the term 'partnerships': 'The most fundamental challenge for individual nations and international agencies in achieving healthy public policy is to encourage collaboration (or developing partnerships) in peace, human rights and social justice, ecology and sustainable development around the globe'.

 Activity 8.4

Take a health issue such as tobacco, alcohol or obesity that is of interest to you and answer the following questions:

1 Which sectors in society and government (local or national) are involved?
2 Identify five or six main influences on your issue, and note for each whether they are a barrier to change or an enabler, and who is involved.
3 Are there conflicts of interest between different parties on your list?
4 Who would the key individuals be if you wanted to bring them together to explore the issue?
5 What would you like to see change and how could you present your goals as achievable and desirable?

 Feedback

Obviously your answer will depend on your issue and your country. For example, if you chose alcohol you may have thought about: the alcohol industry and advertising; the image of alcohol and the way it is promoted to young people; the effects of inner-city regeneration programmes that may have supported the opening of more club and pub venues; problems of policing, violence and demand on accident and emergency services; implications for sexual health; education and its role; and problems with addiction and domestic violence. For each issue, there are key stakeholders you should have listed and considered whether they ever, in your experience, plan services and interventions jointly to address these problems. Given this constellation of issues, have you determined what might be the key goals of change that are required and whether these would be seen as priorities by the different stakeholders?

Summary

You have revised the historical development of health promotion (previously discussed in Chapters 1 and 2) and the emergence of the concept of healthy public policy in the 1980s. You saw how national and international organizations, most notably WHO, have developed the concept of healthy public policy through a series of pronouncements and charters since 1977 and the ongoing discussions, a debate that you can join. In the next chapter, you will learn how healthy public policies can be implemented.

References

Draper R (1987) Healthy public policy: a new political challenge, *Health Promotion* 2(3): 217–18
Milio N (1986) Multisectoral policy and health promotion: where to begin?, *Health Promotion* 1(2): 129–32
World Health Organization (1981) *Global Strategy for Health for All by the Year 2000*. Geneva: WHO
World Health Organization (1984) *Health Promotion: A Discussion Document on the Concept and Principles*. Copenhagen: WHO Regional Office for Europe
World Health Organization (1985) *Targets for Health for All*. Copenhagen: WHO Regional Office for Europe
World Health Organization (1986) *Ottawa Charter for Health Promotion*. Geneva: WHO
World Health Organization (1988) *The Adelaide Recommendations: Healthy Public Policy*. Copenhagen: WHO Regional Office for Europe

9 | Implementing healthy public policy through partnerships

Overview

In this chapter, you will learn how people's needs do not fit neatly within a single agency's responsibilities. Needs are sometimes complex and partnerships are the best way of putting together new and better solutions. Such partnerships may be based around an issue (such as teenage pregnancy), a target group (such as young men), a locality (such as a housing estate), or a statutory authority (local council or health district).

Learning objectives

By the end of this chapter, you will be better able to:

- **describe how partnerships and inter-sectoral working can be implemented**
- **explain the constraints on inter-sectoral partnerships**

Key terms

Community participation A process by which individuals or groups assume responsibility for health matters of their community.

Inter-sectoral collaboration Collaboration between organizations from different sectors working together to come to joint solutions about problems.

Partnership Brings previously separate organizations into a more durable and pervasive relationship, with full commitment to a common mission.

Introduction

As emphasized in Chapter 8, inter-sectoral collaboration and community participation are essential, and yet until recently little was known about how to achieve these in a practical way. To learn about the processes, the World Health Organization launched the Healthy Cities Project in the 1980s to examine how to put Health for All into practice. Initially, only a handful of cities across Europe were committed but quickly the movement spread, and in the review of its progress in 1990 there were thirty 'official' sites, seventeen national networks and over 400 cities worldwide who were taking similar approaches. The project was particularly successful in accumulating practical knowledge about the strategies and structures needed, and the organizational and managerial processes that were likely to be successful in putting health on the political agenda of cities. Not only that, it recognized that to engage policy makers across the board, it needed to demonstrate real achievements and so many demonstration projects and initiatives were developed, involving local people and energizing the movement by showing what could happen. The idea spread from cities to the appropriate local administrative bodies where health and other relevant functions were organized. Called healthy alliances, coalitions or partnerships in different parts of the world, they are seen as ways of putting together new and better solutions to problems that single agencies cannot solve by themselves.

Inter-sectoral partnerships

Partnerships don't just happen and they don't always run smoothly. Few workers at any level have had a great deal of experience in multi-sectoral working. This brings its own challenges of understanding others' points of view, compromise and conflict resolution.

Activity 9.1

What do you think might be the main obstacles to inter-sectoral partnerships?

Feedback

Most people are trained in a single discipline in an agency and adopt the norms and mores of that sector. National policy and resourcing often filter down to local level in vertical streams, making it hard for workers to be flexible with their use of budgets and having to assess their performance in contradictory ways. The more collaborative that healthy public policy is at national level, the easier it is for partnerships to be innovative and responsive to local needs and to deploy resources accordingly. But nothing is ever perfect, and partnership working is the skill of juggling information and priorities to get the best match of service delivery with health need.

Experience of working in partnerships has demonstrated that there are key factors or characteristics that make a partnership effective. The following extract is taken from *The Working Partnership* (Markwell *et al.*, 2003) – an assessment and development tool produced after extensive European research and testing.

 Effective partnerships

Partnerships come in all shapes, sizes and structures. There are no unique models for successful partnerships. Different kinds of partnerships will be effective under different conditions, according to local needs and circumstances, but there are factors that are common to all successful partnerships.

A growing body of evidence from inter-agency and collaborative practice has led to improved understanding of the factors that make partnerships more effective. Analysis of effective partnership working (Audit Commission, 1998; Pratt et al., 1998) show that these factors are centred on the following elements:

- *Leadership and vision* – the management and development of a shared, realistic vision for the partnership's work through the creation of common goals. Effective leadership is demonstrated by influencing, communicating with and motivating others, so that responsibility for decision-making is shared between partners.
- *Organisation and involvement* – the participation of all key local players and, particularly the involvement of communities as equal partners. Not everyone can make the same contribution. Most voluntary organisations are small and locally based, with few staff. They may need resources and time to enable them to become fully engaged.
- *Strategy development and co-ordination* – the development of a clear, community focussed strategy covering the full range of issues supported by relevant policies, plans, objectives, targets, delivery mechanisms and processes. Development of local priorities for action will rely on the assessment of local needs, sharing of data, and a continuing dialogue between partners.
- *Learning and development* – effective partnerships will not only invest in shared objectives and joint outcomes, but will also add value through secondments and other opportunities to share learning and contribute to professional and organisational development in partner organisations. Willingness to listen and learn from each other builds trust.
- *Resources* – the contribution and shared utilisation of information, financial, human and technical resources. The new freedoms to pool budgets and to provide integrated services for example between primary care and social services, can remove some of the traditional barriers to joint working. Cooperation can start by resourcing what everyone wants, for example IT skills training.
- *Evaluation and review* – assessing the quality of the partnership process and measuring progress towards meeting objectives. Partnerships need to demonstrate that they are making a difference and that meetings are more than just talking shops. They must also be able to show that they are making real improvements to services.

Central government has an important role in driving change but partnerships also need the flexibility to reflect local circumstances and resources. It is easy to underestimate the challenges of working together. Partnerships must establish legitimacy in the eyes of local people and enable voluntary sector, community and user groups to participate fully. They must also engage middle managers and frontline staff within statutory agencies.

Partnerships must also devise effective cross-organisational arrangements that can cope with multiple lines of accountability to produce genuine collaborative working. They also need to generate meaningful yet realistic targets for change, and to demonstrate achievements and improvements.

These are formidable challenges that will require long-term commitment. There are a number of barriers to overcome in getting a range of agencies and groups with different responsibilities, structures, systems and cultures to collaborate. Some partnerships, particularly those with a history of working together, may find it easier than others to develop a sustained partnership capable of addressing some of these more complex, longer-term issues. Sustained partnerships take time and demand considerable skills from individuals and organisations. It is one thing to set up partnerships to join things up. It is another to develop the mix of skills, energy and commitment to make partnerships effective.

Key elements for successful partnership

The following list of key elements is taken from the same publication. These are presented with a series of detailed questions for partnership teams to use to assess and improve their ways of working.

Leadership

Effective leadership involves attention to:

- developing and communicating a shared *vision*
- embodying and promoting ownership of and *commitment* to the partnership and its goals
- being alert to factors and *relationships* in the external environment that might affect the partnership

Organization

Clear and effective systems are need for:

- public *participation* in partnership processes and decision making
- *flexibility* in working arrangements
- transparent and effective *management* of the partnership
- *communication* in ways and at times that can be easily understood, interpreted and acted upon

Strategy

The partnership needs to implement its mission and vision via a clear strategy informed by local communities and other stakeholders which focuses on:

- *strategic development* to agree priorities and define outcome targets
- sharing *information and evaluation* of progress and achievements
- a continuous process of *action and review*

Learning

Partner organizations need to attract, manage and develop people to release their full knowledge and potential by:

- *valuing people* as a primary resource
- development and application of *knowledge and skills*
- supporting *innovation*

Resources

The contribution and shared utilization of resources, including

- building and strengthening *social capital* (which you will learn about in Chapter 10)
- managing and pooling *financial resources*

- making *information* work
- using information and communication *technology* appropriately

Programmes

Partners seek to develop coordinated programmes and integrated services that fit together well. This requires attention to:

- realizing added value from joint *planning*
- focused *delivery*
- regular *monitoring* and review

 Activity 9.2

Building on the example you thought about in Activity 8.4, how would you organize a partnership to address the issue you described? Who would be on it and why? In the role of convenor, how would you organize the first few meetings? What would be the important things to do first?

 Feedback

You should have noted key stakeholders for your chosen issue, whose activities would potentially have an influence on those aspects of health you were looking for. However, when it comes to mobilizing these forces locally, it is not always so easy to identify the relevant individuals who have responsibility for service delivery and control over resources. In the example of alcohol, the local police and Accident and Emergency services would be identifiable, but who would you involve to represent the alcohol industry locally? Whoever you have identified and invited to an initial meeting, partnership working requires that you understand the different positions and concerns that people bring to the table. Giving time to sharing information about the issue, listening to the views of partners about the constraints they may be operating under, or the barriers to change they face, is important. You need to value people's contributions and discuss the opportunities for change so as to come to an initial agreed, achievable goal. Sometimes these first steps may fall short of what you would want to achieve eventually, but they will build the basis of further work and create an atmosphere of trust and shared ownership. Agreeing processes of working, how often to meet, what further information can be shared, who else to involve, all will be important groundwork for partnership working.

Healthy public policy in the twenty-first century

While the enthusiastic advocates of health promotion in the 1980s seemed to have solutions to solve the world's problems, health promoters still need to convince others outside the field of health promotion. There has been substantial progress towards an understanding of healthy public policy in countries around the world, even if it is not fully implemented. To some extent, in some countries it has become almost the norm. Policies are to a large extent integrated or at least aligned and are focused on reducing inequity. The rising cost of health care coupled with the increased demands from an ageing society with increasing expectations has encouraged governments to see the necessity of focusing on health.

In the UK, for example, action on inequalities and inter-sectoral working has been placed centrally and partnerships, principally between health and local authorities, have become necessary parts of the public sector delivery system. Actions and indicators of progress across government departments focus on four areas: supporting families, mothers and children; engaging communities and individuals; preventing illness and providing effective treatment and care; and addressing the underlying determinants of health. A new target for a reduction in inequalities in health (which had been rising since the 1970s) was set to reduce inequalities in infant mortality and life expectancy at birth by 10 per cent by 2010. However, public health policy may yet put the emphasis back on individual responsibility and health care but at least there is greater cross-government understanding, some shifting of resources and significant changes throughout the health system.

In France, the High Committee on Public Health (2003) set out a detailed framework for action to control the increasing cost of health care. The Committee stated that health policy needs to cover three levels: (1) at the level of factors that determine health in order to promote good health; (2) to ensure top quality care is available when needed; and (3) rehabilitation. The authors state: 'Although this holistic idea is sometimes alluded to in an abstract fashion in France, rarely is anything concrete done about it. Resources and attention are massively concentrated at the second level of attention i.e. care and treatment. Ever since the end of the Second World War, policy has focussed on improving access to health care rather than improving health'. So while this system is at an early stage of developing healthy public policy, the understanding and evidence are growing.

Sweden has taken it a stage further than most countries. The Swedish National Institute for Public Health announced aims to create the conditions for good health on equal terms for the entire population (Agren, 2003). The new Public Health Policy aims to create the conditions for good health on equal terms for the entire population, recognizing that politicians cannot prevent deaths and illness, but can influence what lies behind (i.e. the upstream approach). The eleven general objectives (Table 9.1) give an indication of the priority placed on the living and working conditions (social, economic and environmental determinants) rather than the health goals. Indeed, they have recast their health targets as indicators of progress of achievement in addressing the determinants rather than as goals in themselves.

Table 9.1 Sweden's eleven public health objectives

1	Participation and influence in society
2	Economic and social security
3	Secure and favourable conditions during childhood and adolescence
4	Healthier working life
5	Healthy and safe environments and products
6	Health and medical care that more actively promotes good health
7	Effective protection against communicable diseases
8	Safe sexuality and good productive health
9	Increased physical activity
10	Good eating habits and safe food
11	Reduced use of tobacco and alcohol, a society free from illicit drugs and doping and a reduction in the harmful effects of excessive gambling

Source: Agren (2003)

 Activity 9.3

Keeping with the example you used in Activity 9.2, look at the way these goals emphasize the wider determinants of health. Try recasting the aims of your 'partnership' in 'upstream' terms. What difference does that make to the partnership and its objectives?

 Feedback

Up to now, your objectives have probably been couched in terms of reducing illness or accidents, supporting a change in individual behaviour, perhaps reorganizing the way services are delivered. When your issue is looked at from the perspective of participation and influence in society, economic and social security, and secure and favourable conditions during childhood and adolescence, it should become clear that there are fundamental and common objectives across all sectors that influence health. So, access to good living conditions, education and employment, for example, all have a bearing on health in its broader sense. Recognizing these underlying determinants in inter-sectoral working enables different sectors to work to a common purpose, even when their individual objectives may appear to differ, and emphasizes the need for common overarching policy objectives that all can sign up to.

Finally, the World Health Organization has launched an initiative to place even further emphasis on the importance of governments investing in the social and economic determinants of health. So while earlier models focused on environmental determinants and on the potential health impacts of decisions made in different sectors, the 'Investment for Health and Development' approach challenges the emphasis on investment in health care at the expense of investment in jobs, social conditions and education, based on the evidence of where most health can effectively be 'bought' in society. This goes well beyond traditional inter-sectoral health promotion programmes to challenge resource distribution and examine whole-systems approaches. Importantly, it draws in the economic sector, not just public spending, to which most previous healthy public policy approaches have by and large been excluded (WHO, 2002).

Summary

You have learned about healthy public policy and how health promotion needs to be involved in the policy process both within and beyond the health sector. Healthy public policy is important for health promotion because so many of the factors that influence health lie outside the remit of the health sector or individuals' behaviour. Inter-sectoral (partnership) working is fundamental to achieving integrated healthy public policy.

References

Agren G (2003) *Sweden's New Public Health Policy*. Stockholm: Swedish National Institute for Public Health
Audit Commission (1998) *A Fruitful Partnership: Effective Partnership Working*. London: Audit Commission
High Committee on Public Health (2003) *Health in France 2002*. Paris: John Libbey Eurotext
Markwell S, Watson J, Speller V *et al.* (2003) *The Working Partnership – Book 1*. London: Health Development Agency
Pratt J, Plamping D, Gordon P (1998) *Partnership: Fit for Purpose?* London: King's Fund
World Health Organization (2002) *Investment for Health: A Discussion of the Role of Economic and Social Determinants*. Copenhagen: WHO Regional Office for Europe

10 | Working with communities

Overview

As you will have already seen, community participation is a central tenet of the Health for All strategy and the Ottawa Charter, and a defining principle of health promotion. While health promotion can and does act on individuals, what distinguishes it from individual preventive care is a focus on creating the conditions for change in individuals and groups at the community level. In this chapter, you will explore the ways in which health promoters work with communities to improve their health. You will look at the definitions of the concepts of community, community participation, empowerment, community development and social capital and briefly examine some of the methods and approaches to working successfully with communities.

Learning objectives

After working through this chapter, you will be better able to:

- understand key concepts, principles and the history of community development in health
- describe practical approaches to working with communities and issues of evaluating community development work
- appreciate the differing perspectives and constraints on working with communities, both from the view point of community members and professionals

Key terms

Community A neighbourhood and/or group with common interests and identity

Community development The process of change in neighbourhoods and communities. It aims to increase the extent and effectiveness of community action, community activity and agencies' relationships with communities.

Empowerment A central tenet of health promotion, whereby individuals are given knowledge, skills and opportunity to develop a sense of control and mastery over life circumstances.

Social capital Facets such as sociability, social networks, trust, reciprocity and community and civic engagement.

What is a community?

Although the meaning of community may appear self-evident, it is a concept that has defied simple definition. The most obvious type of community is one defined by geography, a district in a town, an estate or neighbourhood, or a school – but such a community is not homogeneous. It consists of people of different ages, ethnicities, interests and aspirations. So community can also be defined by interest group, health and social need, political views, and so on. Laverack (2004) identifies four key characteristics of community:

- a spatial dimension, i.e. a place or locale
- non-spatial dimensions (interests, issues, identities) that involve people who otherwise make up heterogeneous and disparate groups
- social interactions that are dynamic and bind people into relationships with one another
- identification of shared needs and concerns that can be achieved through a process of collective action

As you look more at the principles of working with communities, you will see that some of the key issues relate to notions of power and control in the relationship between community members and professionals planning and providing services for them. Thus in working with communities, an understanding of who the community comprises and why they have a common or shared need is essential. So too is the recognition that communities can only define themselves.

 Activity 10.1

Using the four categories above, list the different communities that you feel part of. Think then about a family member or close friend. Do they belong to the same communities? Do they interact with other groups?

 Feedback

You may have thought about the following types of community:

- where you live – street, village or town
- your hobbies or leisure activities – for example, you may belong to a sports club
- your colleagues at work or professional body
- perhaps you belong to a political group such as an environmental conservation group

So people 'belong' to a number of different communities at any one time and define their 'membership' themselves. A single community, although sharing many attributes, is not homogeneous.

What is community development?

The following extract by Henderson and colleagues (2004), on the definition of community development and its history, points out the importance of understanding the key events and turning points in the history of community development and enables a comparison of approaches. They also provide some models and ways of thinking about the essential principles and aims of community development.

 Activity 10.2

While reading it, note the different perspectives from different sectors or professional groups as regards: (1) their ideas of power and control over people and life circumstances; (2) the drive for social change; and (3) the different types of participation that it encompasses.

 Defining community development

Community development seeks to bring about change locally, regionally and nationally. People differ on the definition of community development and the term is constantly under review. There are, however, some essential baselines. Community development is not just about what happens in neighbourhoods and interest groups: it is also concerned with how organisations and agencies respond to community issues and how they support local initiatives. One way of defining community development is to set out its goals. These are: to combat social exclusion; to promote participation; and to encourage people to acquire new skills.

The Standing Conference for Community Development's (SCCD 2001) framework for community development summarised some of the core values and commitments of community development and provides a useful basis to work from. The SCCD stated: 'Community development is about building active and sustainable communities based on social justice and mutual respect. It is about changing power structures to remove the barriers that prevent people from participating in the issues that affect their lives. Community workers support individuals, groups and organisations in this process on the basis of the following values and commitments:

Values
- Social justice: enabling people to claim their human rights, meet their needs and have greater control over the decision-making processes that affect their lives.
- Participation: facilitating democratic involvement by people in the issues which affect their lives based on full citizenship, autonomy and shared power, skills, knowledge and experience.
- Equality: challenging the attitudes of individuals and the practices of institutions and society, which discriminate against, and marginalise, people.

- Learning: recognising the skills, knowledge and expertise that people contribute and develop by taking action to tackle social, economic, political and environmental problems.
- Cooperation: working together to identify and implement action, based on mutual respect of diverse cultures and contributions.

Commitments
- Challenging discrimination and oppressive practices within organisations, institutions and communities.
- Developing practice and policy that protects the environment.
- Encouraging networking and connections between communities and organisations.
- Ensuring access and choice for all groups and individuals within society.
- Influencing policy and programmes from the perspective of communities.
- Prioritising the issues of concern to people experiencing poverty and social exclusion.
- Promoting social change that is long-term and sustainable.
- Reversing inequality and the imbalance of power relationships in society.
- Supporting community-led collective action.

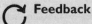 **Feedback**

Community development works at different levels, on individuals in communities, and on organizations and the structure of society. From the perspective of the individual, and those working at the front line supporting them, it emphasizes empowerment, helping people learn new skills and understanding, and supporting people to challenge aspects of their lives that affect their health and ability to function. At the organizational level, it requires politicians and leaders to understand how their actions affect individuals and the need to be aware of community views. Structurally, it means that services and systems become more open to community members so that they have a voice and can influence them. This means professionals giving up some of their control over decision making and sharing power with community members. Practically, this requires establishing ways of allowing the community access to decision-making processes through active participation at all levels, from individual interactions with service providers to involvement in service planning and funding decisions.

The building blocks of community development

A different approach is to think of the aims of community development in terms of building blocks, or core dimensions. This is how the Scottish Community Development Centre sets about the task. Four of the building blocks are about community empowerment; the other five are called 'quality-of-life' building blocks because they indicate the sort of community that community development tries to achieve. In Table 10.1, the first of each pair of statements is a statement of process (the action); the second is a statement of outcome. The core dimensions of community development are like a pyramid. These dimensions provide clear guidelines for defining community development. They also encourage practitioners and

Table 10.1 Building blocks for community development

Process	Outcome
Community empowerment	
Personal empowerment	A learning community
Positive action	A fair and just community
Community organizing and volunteer support	An active and organized community
Participation and involvement	An influential community
Quality of life	
Community economic development	A shared wealth
Social and service development	A caring community
Community environmental action	A safe and healthy community
Community arts and cultural development	A creative community
Governance and development	A citizens' community

Source: Barr and Hashagen (2000)

others to adapt them to their own values and settings, and to use them as building blocks. The core dimensions are used throughout the UK, chiefly as a part of an evaluation model for community development.

Another way of looking at community development is to distinguish between aspects concerned with the group of people being worked with and those concerned with the worker – the characteristics and approach of the person doing the work (Table 10.2).

Principles for involving the public

These are described by Crowley (2000). They include:

- The community is an asset and part of the solution, not the problem.
- Community representatives need support to link to the wider community and their input must be accountable to the local community.
- Any approach must involve marginalized minority groups – people with sensory or physical disability, gay men and lesbians, minority ethnic groups, etc.
- Financial support is necessary to ensure access – for a crèche, carer support, interpretation (including sign language, translation, audiotapes, etc.).
- Community participation strategies are required where the community can set the agenda and raise issues that are of concern to them.
- To involve the public, statutory bodies need to be developed so that they are responsive to the community's view.
- The process is important because if the community does not see some results from their voluntary involvement, they will lose interest.
- If meetings include local people they must be conducted in a way as to ensure their participation, such as by avoiding jargon.

Table 10.2 Group aspects versus worker aspects

Group aspects	Worker aspects
Felt needs The needs that people want to work with are their own felt and expressed needs	**Collectivization** Making problems collective that initially, individuals may perceive as their own
Personal responsibility Community development is committed to people doing things for themselves and taking personal responsibility for them, not having things done for or to them	**Participation** The community development worker is interested in promoting participatory forms of membership and decision making
Personal experience and need A community group is made up of people who have experienced at first hand the problems which led to setting up that group and who will benefit from its work	**Partnership** This refers to how a worker relates to a group – conveyed in such phrases as 'working with people and not for them' and 'start where people are at'. The worker does not seek to lead groups, or use them to pursue his or her own ends
Voluntary Involvement is voluntary, not required by legal or administrative rules	**Process** Promoting confidence, skills, knowledge and consciousness in those who take part in group activities and action
Constituency The community development work will benefit a wider constituency than just those involved in a group, and will perhaps benefit the wider community	**Task** Supporting a group to achieve agreed objectives and outcomes
	Perspective Helping local people to understand the reasons for external problems

Source: Thomas (1983)

 Activity 10.3

> The following short history of community development is adapted from Henderson *et al.* (2004) and describes the tensions or conflicts that exist between different perspectives. To help you make these rather theoretical statements more real, pick an issue of relevance to you and make notes as to how it may be acted upon and perceived from these different standpoints.

📖 A short history of community development

This historical perspective is based on the themes:

*   Changing champions
*   Generalist versus specialist
*   Voluntary, community and statutory sectors
*   Internationalism
*   Social movement/profession
*   Conservatism/radicalism.

Changing champions

Community development has only rarely existed in its own right. It has needed the backing of established professions. The education field has supported community associations (particularly in the inter-war period), youth and community work and community-based adult education. During the late 1960s to late 1970s, social work was the main sponsor of community development, later developing community social work. Economic development and regeneration is the most recent backer of community development, supporting community enterprises and increasingly engaging with the community in partnerships.

From the mid-1980s, social work virtually stopped sponsoring community development. Education maintained a role in Scotland, but overall regeneration has been the main player. Some other areas have become interested in community development: public health, housing and community arts. One effect of changing champions is that community development has had to survive with a very weak infrastructure – that is, the membership, training and support organisations that it needs to sustain itself.

Generalist v specialist

There is a tension or struggle within community development between those who see it as having a core body of values, knowledge and skills which permeate other professions (specialist); and those who see it as a malleable concept which can be adjusted to fit particular circumstances (generalist). The tension has often been creative. Examples of the specialist school of thought are:

*   The work of the settlements at the end of the 19th century (a significant point of origin for community development)
*   The United Nations' use of the concept in the 1950s
*   Community development in the new towns and on council estates after World War II
*   The report *Community work and social change* (Gulbenkian Foundation, 1968)
*   The Home Office Community Development Projects (1968–77)
*   The policies of the umbrella organization for community development – the Standing Conference for Community Development.

Examples of the generalist school are:

*   The Colonial Service's use of community development
*   Youth work during the 1970s
*   Community social work and community probation work (1970s–1980s)
*   Community health projects
*   Environmental action
*   Drugs prevention work.

Voluntary, community and statutory sectors

In the UK, until the publication of the Seebohm Report (1968) on community work in social services departments, the voluntary sector was the driving force behind community development, often under the leadership of charismatic individuals. There was some anxiety that the experience of the Community Development Projects, which put forward a radical analysis of the causes of poverty in the communities where they were based, would result in statutory organizations losing interest in community development. This anxiety proved unfounded. The voluntary sector is still a key player. In some rural areas, for example, rural community councils rather than local authorities are still the main community development organisations. Over the past 20 years, local authorities and health authorities have demonstrated an increasing commitment to community development. The statutory sector, directly or indirectly, is the main funder of community development, drawing on government and European grants. Research in the early 1990s, by the Community Development Foundation, revealed the existence of a community sector alongside the more established voluntary sector. Using 'community sector' to refer to those organisations which are generally smaller and have no staff has proved a useful shorthand. It is now common to refer to the community sector as well as the voluntary sector.

Internationalism

During the 1970s and 1980s, practice and theory in the USA had a significant influence on community development thinking. This has since waned. The writings of Paulo Freire, the Brazilian educationalist, have been a consistent influence, on ideas if not on practice. His most notable work is *Pedagogy of the Oppressed* (Freire, 1972). It is no accident that the National Training Organisation, set up in the U.K. in 1999, for community work, adult education, youth work and community education, was named PAULO. As in the health sector, there have been active community development links between high and low income countries for a number of years. Development agencies such as Oxfam have helped to exchange practice and participatory action research.

Social movement/profession

It is important to be aware that the origins of community development lie in social movements, as well as in professions. In the U.K., the squatting movement at the end of the 1960s was one of the more striking examples of a social movement that saw itself as being part of community development. This was followed by widespread opposition to slum clearance, inner-city redevelopment, road-building schemes and, more recently, environmental hazards. There are also elements of social movement in smaller-scale activities: for example, demands made by residents for safe play areas for children. The social movement and professional elements of community development are not necessarily in conflict. Both have driven community development forward and arguably they need each other. The energies and commitment of local people are the lifeblood of community development and most social movements need, at some point, to develop more formal organisations. There has been a growing awareness that community development must avoid becoming trapped – literally and metaphorically – at the neighbourhood level. If change is to occur, work has to be done within key organisations and agencies. Over the past 20 years there have been examples of local authorities using resources for community development for policy work, as well as for practice. Most people in community development see the importance of this.

Conservatism/radicalism

Conservative and radical ideas interweave through the history of community development. Two major examples are feminist and black perspectives. Both of these movements criticized community development for failing to engage with key issues and for being too conservative. Equally, many of those in disability organisations argue that they have done more than community development workers to involve users in policy making. Some organisations want to use community development as a tool for putting particular policies and programmes into practice; others want to use it to challenge assumptions, policies and resource allocations. Given the structure and identity of community development, we should not be surprised that its history is characterised by competing viewpoints.

 Feedback

Whatever the issue you thought about while reading this extract, it should have become apparent that viewed from the different standpoints – professional, voluntary sector group, individual, etc. – there is the potential for creative tension, rather than conflict. Although different professional groups may have 'owned' community development approaches in the past, and it has been associated with political movements and struggle for social change, the commitment to 'working with communities' and valuing their perspective is embedded in the policy and practice of many sectors nowadays. However, community development will always be diverse in its methods, and have to attend to *both* working with individuals and groups, *and* workers and organizational processes – at the same time. It is by addressing this potential conflict and creating solutions, that both the needs of individuals and those of the wider society can be addressed. That is the essence of community development.

Empowerment

The concept of empowerment is embodied in the Ottawa Charter in the phrase 'enabling people to take control over and to improve their health' (WHO, 1986). There are (at least) two rather differing perspectives on empowerment that influence health promotion practice today: the critical consciousness raising perspective of Freire (1972) and the psychological construct of self-efficacy (Bandura, 1977). Freire, working in Brazil in the 1950s and 1960s, sought through education to liberate people from the oppression of poverty and their associated helplessness to change the circumstances of their lives. The process of critical consciousness raising 'refers to learning to perceive social, political, and economic contradictions and to take action against the oppressive elements of reality' (Freire, 1972). It is inextricably related to notions of sharing power, as Freire puts it, carrying out transformations *with* the oppressed rather than *for* them. Freire's work has been influential in health education theory as it is centred around the acquisition of information and knowledge to bring about change and emphasizes the power of collective social action.

Self-efficacy relates to individuals' self-perceptions of their competence at performing particular activities (Bandura, 1977). It differs from self-esteem, which is a rather more global concept of feelings of self-worth, in that self-efficacy is situation specific. Individuals can feel control or mastery over certain behaviours, while avoiding activities that they feel exceed their coping capacities. Community development approaches have the potential to both empower through raising individuals' beliefs in their own capabilities – either to make personal behaviour changes or to participate more fully in collective activities (such as having the confidence to speak up at meetings, for example) – and through working with groups to achieve social change by advocacy and facilitating engagement with decision makers. The Building Blocks of Community Development (Barr and Hashagen, 2000) include personal empowerment, community organizing and positive action as key elements of community empowerment. In the descriptions of workers' responsibilities, the roles of promoting confidence, skills, knowledge and consciousness in those who take part in group activities and action all result in individual and community empowerment.

Community participation

Community participation is used sometimes interchangeably with community development. In fact, it is a more general term and can be used to describe different forms and degrees of involvement, which are usually considered to relate to different levels of sharing power between communities and decision makers. Arnstein's (1971) ladder of participation is the classic description of these different levels (Table 10.3).

While climbing up the ladder has been considered the goal of increasing degrees of empowerment and control, it must be remembered that not all communities, or individuals within a community, wish to have total control, or even significant responsibility. For some aspects of working with communities, simply provision of information may be appropriate, or working in mutually respectful partnerships of community members and professionals. At all times, the key issues are: What is the purpose of the work? To what extent do the community want to be involved? Are those who are engaged in activities actually representing the community, or engaging in their own personal desire for increased power, perhaps resulting in the further exclusion of marginalized groups? What are the goals of the health and social workers and is their style of working empowering?

Table 10.3 Arnstein's ladder of participation

Degrees of actual power	Control
	Delegated power
	Partnership
Degrees of tokenism	Placation
	Consultation
	Informing
Non-participation	Therapy
	Manipulation

Source: Arnstein (1971)

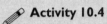

Activity 10.4

Read the following two descriptions of community development activity from Ron Labonte (1996). For each think about the dimensions of empowerment, degrees of participation, and professional roles indicated.

 Community development: two examples

In La Casa Dona Juana, a social space for Latin American women in Toronto, participants identify the different skills or 'gifts' that individual members bring to the collective and to its activities. Women who are skilled in writing prepare the grant applications, and teach other women in the process. Women who are skilled in cooking take a leadership role in the collective kitchen, and pass skills on to other women during the process. Women who are skilled in budgeting plan the menus or purchases for the collectives, again transferring their knowledge to other collective members. Women who are skilled in sewing techniques take leadership in the sewing collective. In the 'outside' world, budgeting and grant-writing skills may be highly valued, and those who have them may be given more social status and power over others. But in La Casa Dona Juana, due partly to the feminist organizing beliefs of the health and social service professionals who provided the space and resources to start it, budgeting and grants writing are merely one set of social skills no more or less important than those involved in cooking, menu-planning or sewing . . .

Maori people in Aotearoa, New Zealand suffer in the same ways that other indigenous colonized people suffer. Many of them are poor, unemployed, victimized and self-victimizing with alcohol and abuse. Sympathetic Pakeha (as Maori refer to others) go to great lengths to decry the powerlessness and impoverishment that create their poor health. They want to focus attention on what we now call the 'determinants of health', poverty, pollution, discrimination, all of which are effects of a social system whose dominant paradigm is power-over. Pakeha health workers do not want to blame poor Maori health on their high smoking rates, poor nutrition habits, bad-parenting skills or lack of family planning. But to many Maori, this explanation is little better than the lifestyle victim-blaming it replaces. While they lack the legislative authority to reorganize their communities as autonomous political systems, many Maori are doing so anyway. In one instance, they used government funds for a computer training programme for unemployed youth to develop their own census of every Maori woman, man and child. Their intention is to keep tabs on the individuals in their communities. When a person begins to run into difficulties, counsellors and healers from their extended families can act to re-integrate them in ways that are more in keeping with Maori culture. The Maori leaders who developed this programme were asked 'How can you do this? Only elected governments can create such a census. You don't have the authoriy or the power to do this.' They replied, 'We act as if we have the authority and the power. And in acting this way, we develop the very authority and power you say we do not possess.' There is even a name for this stance: tino rangitiratanga, or 'acting from the position of Maori chieftaincy', more commonly defined as Maori self-determination, or what we would call power-from-within.

Feedback

The sorts of issues you should have noted may include:

1 In La Casa Dona Juana, the women were empowered through having their self-efficacy increased through acknowledgment and practice of individual skills and by no skill being valued above another. Their sense of control and additional confidence was increased as they taught their skills to others, and by taking leadership roles. Participation appeared equally shared between members and workers, who took supportive and facilitative roles. The collective was run by the members, but the workers had initially used their power to access resources and facilities to establish it, but then appear to have relinquished control.

2 In Aotearoa, the Maori empowered themselves through accessing training to increase their skills. They did not trust the professionals' analysis of their problems, as they felt this did not address their current individual health needs, whether or not determinants of health were improved. They took control of information that belonged to them, with the agreement of the whole community, and organized relevant services. Through this they took control and power, rather than having it delegated to them. The professionals did not seem to be listening to the needs and wishes of the community, and appeared satisfied with token degrees of participation.

Social capital

Social capital is a concept related to community development but it is not the same thing. It has grown out of the recognition of the positive impact on health of social support and social ties to the community through participation and involvement in social networks. There has been more recent interest in ways of 'building social capital', to increase the health-promoting capacities of communities and their resilience to negative influences on health. It is described clearly in the following extract from Swann and Morgan (2002).

 Activity 10.5

While reading the following extract, think about the similarities and differences between social capital and community development.

 What is social capital?

Over the last ten years, the notion that social, psychological, economic and contextual factors impact significantly on the health of individuals and communities has gained in currency as the evidence base has grown. At the same time, individual models of health behaviours and outcomes have declined in popularity and use within public health and health promotion. Within this context, the concept of social capital has emerged as having potential to further articulate the relationship between health and its broader determinants. Social capital can be broadly described as the resources within a community that create family and social organisation. These resources, which arise out of activities such as civic engagement, social support or participation, benefit individuals, but are developed in relationship to and with others, for example within groups or communities. Key constructs within the concept, often – and variously – used as indicators, include social relationships, group membership, shared norms, trust, formal and informal social networks, reciprocity and civic engagement.

Social capital is not an entirely novel concept. It has roots in the work of sociologists such as Durkheim, whose work on group life led to the proposition that involvement and support was the solution to anomie and suicide, and William Julius Wilson, who studied the role of social isolation in the lives and futures of inner-city 'urban-underclass' residents. Its current popularity can be traced to work by Robert Putnam (1993) on civic engagement in Italy. Putnam investigated social capital in Italy by taking measures of a number of indicators, including levels of memberships of clubs/societies, time spent socialising, time spent in reciprocal activities, beliefs/norms about the intentions of others (trust), and the extent of friendship networks. He suggests that a number of factors are responsible for the erosion of social capital in deprived areas, including lack of time, poverty, residential mobility, suburbanisation, disruption of family ties, and changes in economic structure. Campbell et al. (1999) give the following as examples of characteristics of communities where social capital is abundant:

- Individuals feel an obligation to help others and those in need, represented through dense personal networks of support that link individuals, households and peer groups.
- There is willingness and capacity to make use of community resources, notably those provided by the state, evidenced for example in use of institutionalized health service systems.
- Individuals exhibit more trust and less fear in interacting with others in the community, manifested for example in positive attitudes towards personal interactions, use of community facilities, sense of 'belonging' to the community.

The relationship between social capital and health

But what is the link between social capital and health? In general, populations with high levels of material deprivation and poverty have worse health. For example, Kawachi (1996) found, in prospective studies of professional men in the US, that those with the lowest level of social networks were significantly more likely to die of cardiovascular disease. Cooper et al. (1999) found that women living in UK neighbourhoods which they perceived to be high in elements of social capital were less likely to smoke, after controlling for material deprivation and socio-economic factors. Campbell et al. suggest that some elements of Putnam's original concept of social capital (particularly trust and civic engagement) might be more health enhancing than others. In this study, communities and networks were found to be more complex and multi-layered than those defined by geographical boundaries such as street or ward, and strong differences within communities were found in the way that elements of social capital were created, sustained and accessed. There were also clear differences in the types of community networks that men and women created and drew upon in their day-to-day lives, and in the type of support they gave and received from these networks. Individual constructions of health and relations to community appeared to vary according to gender, ethnicity and life-stage. These findings are congruent with broader work on health inequalities, where clear patterns of health outcomes and behaviours by gender, ethnicity, life-stage and income can be observed. Campbell et al. (1999) have suggested that high levels of social capital may act as a buffer in deprived communities, serving to shield them from some of the worst effects of deprivation. Others have made the link between deprivation and health via the psychological constructs of self-efficacy and stress, with those lowest on socio-economic scales having least control over their life and work environments, more stress, and subsequently worse health.

↻ Feedback

You may have noted that both social capital and community development refer to communities as multi-layered and heterogeneous; that both refer to involvement in groups and civic society – participating actively being central. Both are related to the reduction of inequalities in health and a positive sense of health and well-being. However, there are key differences. Social capital refers to the capacity of communities and the networks that exist within and between groups, without necessarily any reference to state institutions, professional relationships or social action for change. Different dimensions of social capital provide the means for measuring attributes of the healthiness of a community – the aspects that community development may be trying to enhance. So community development is a process that has goals of empowerment and change, some of which may be measured by the types of indicator that social capital encompasses. Social capital is a useful construct that endeavours to describe with greater clarity fuzzy concepts like empowerment and the notion of an enabled community that has some degree of control over local circumstance.

Ways of working with communities

Henderson et al. (2004) provide some practical details and exercises to enable workers to profile their community and understand its perceived needs and assets. They emphasize the importance of looking at its strengths and resources – that is, its social capital. A review of the research literature on participatory approaches in health promotion and health planning showed that the two most common methods used are participatory action research and rapid appraisals (Rifkin et al., 2000). Participatory action research, which has its origins in the work of Freire, involves all those concerned with the research outcomes (that is, researchers, professional and community members) participating equally at all stages in the planning, information collection and interpretation of results. Rapid appraisals have more recently become popular in the health and development fields. The features of both are similar but rapid appraisals are more usually done to inform planning and service issues.

Good practice guidelines

Finally, have a look at the good practice guidelines below about the best ways to involve the community in health. This comes from a review of over 200 community participation projects in England in the late 1990s, working with diverse communities on a wide range of health issues. This provides a clear and practical checklist of actions for working with communities that reflects all that has been learnt from work on empowerment, social action and community development. The main good practice issues are grouped under five main headings.

Clear and realistic role and remit

Good practice requires:

- projects to work within a wide definition of health and to establish health as an important community issue
- clarity and consensus about participatory principles and values and their implications
- community participation at all stages of a project's development and work
- changes in the culture and ways of working of the statutory sector
- a realistic remit for community projects and initiatives based on the time and resources available and the needs and history of the community/users the project is working with
- respect for, and acceptance of, minority/different needs and the need for mainstream as well as specific project work

Adequate and appropriate resources to meet the project remit

Good practice requires:

- secure, adequate and long-term funding
- accessible and appropriate premises
- an experienced, long-term team with community development skills
- reliable, committed and properly supported volunteers/activists

Adequate and appropriate management and evaluation to support the project

Good practice requires:

- effective and supportive project management (be it through a management committee or line management model) by people with appropriate time, skills and experience
- clearly defined structural arrangements between projects and key agencies to avoid too much reliance on individuals and to ensure clear pathways for feeding in community needs and concerns
- community involvement in project management and decision making
- appropriate and adequate monitoring and evaluation to inform project planning and development in ongoing ways

Recognition of the importance of the wider environment within which projects operate

Good practice requires:

- building on the past history and experience of communities and local agencies and developing new projects within that context

- harnessing the political support of local politicians and linking projects to new national policy openings endorsing community participation
- effective inter-agency/sector links and partnership working at both local and district/city-wide levels

Building in long-term sustainability

Good practice requires:

- linking community health projects into the wide and variable agendas for change that are emerging in the health and social policy fields
- projects being able to show real changes/gains they have achieved and to promote these to communities, funders and agencies
- building community capacity in terms of skills, information access points, networks and groups
- organization development to ensure local agencies and professionals have the skills, knowledge and commitment to support the effectiveness of local community participation work, build community needs and views into their planning, policy and priority setting and to respond appropriately to community identified
- seeing sustainability as an integral part of project work, not a final stage

Summary

You have learnt about different concepts of 'community' and of community development as an approach to promote public health. You then saw how three particular concepts – empowerment, community participation, and social capital – have been proposed to explain the way communities may have an impact on people's health. Finally, you learnt about ways of working effectively with communities.

References

Arnstein SR (1971) Eight rungs on the ladder of citizen participation, in Cahn SE, Passett BA (eds.) *Citizen Participation: Effecting Community Change*. New York: Praeger

Bandura A (1977) Self-efficacy: towards a unifying theory of behavioural change, *Psychological Review* 64(2): 191–215

Barr A, Hashagen S (2000) *ABCD Handbook: A Framework for Evaluating Community Development*. London: CDF Publications

Campbell C, Wood R, Kelly M (1999) *Social Capital and Health*. London: Health Education Authority

Cooper H *et al.* (1999) *The Influence of Social Support and Social Capital on Health: A Review and Analysis of British Data*. London: Health Education Authority

Crowley P (2000) Community development and primary care groups, in *Communities Developing for Health*. Liverpool: UK Health for All Network

Freire P (1972) *Pedagogy of the Oppressed*. Harmondsworth: Penguin

Gulbenkian Foundation (1968) *Community Work and Social Change*. London: Longman

Henderson P, Summer S, Raj T (2004) *Developing Healthier Communities: An Introductory Course for People Using Community Development Approaches to Improve Health and Tackle Health Inequalities*. London: Health Development Agency

Kawachi I (1996) A prospective study of social networks in relation to total mortality and cardiovascular disease in the USA, *Journal of Epidemiology and Community Health* 50: 245–91

Labonte R (1996) *Community development in the public health sector: the possibilities of an empowering relationship between the state and civil society*, PhD thesis, York University, Toronto

Laverack G (2004) *Health Promotion Practice: Power and Empowerment*. London: Sage

Putnam R (1993) *Making Democracy Work: Civic Traditions in Modern Italy*. Princeton, NJ: Princeton University Press

Rifkin SB, Lewando-Hundt G, Draper AK (2000) *Participatory Approaches in Health Promotion and Health Planning: A Literature Review*. London: Health Development Agency

Seebohm Report (1968) *Report of the Committee on Local Authority and Allied Personal Social Services* (The Seebohm Report). London: HMSO

Standing Conference for Community Development (2001) *Strategic Framework for Community Development*. Sheffield: SCCD

Swann C, Morgan A (2002) Introduction, in Swann C, Morgan A (eds.) *Social Capital for Health: Insights from Qualitative Research*. London: Health Development Agency

Thomas DN (1983) *The Making of Community Work*. London: George Allen & Unwin

World Health Organization (1986) *The Ottawa Charter for Health Promotion*. Geneva: WHO

Further reading

For more information about methods, see both Henderson *et al.* (2004) and Rifkin *et al.* (2000).

SECTION 4

Implementing health promotion

Risk management, perception and communication in health care

11

Overview

In this chapter, you will learn about a definition of risk followed by a framework for the management of risk, and an overview of risk perception and the cognitive pitfalls present when dealing with risk. It closes with a discussion of risk communication.

Learning objectives

By the end of this chapter, you will be able to:

- **deconstruct risk into its main components**
- **apply management techniques to mitigate the risk**
- **plan how to prepare for risk situations**
- **design strategies on how to communicate in risk situations**

Key terms

Aleatory uncertainty A situation in which you have fairly good knowledge of the probability of a particular outcome as it is known to be random.

Epistemic uncertainty A situation in which you have no knowledge of the probability of a particular outcome.

Heuristics Problem solving by application of a method that generally yields reasonable solutions, as opposed to finding the best one.

Message mapping Achieving message clarity and conciseness based on developing a consensus message platform, providing visual aids and road maps for displaying structurally organized responses to anticipated high concern issues, focused at specific stakeholder groups.

Risk The probability that an event will occur within a specified time.

Risk and risk management

'The real world isn't predictable. Should we consider everything that can happen?' Many situations in health promotion can be seen as an example of decision making in the presence of high risk, involving imperfect information as well as personal preferences, which, at times, can be regarded as inconsistent with rational behaviour. While all of us talk about risk, few of us have a concise understanding of the concept. So, what is risk?

Risk consists of two parts: an undesirable outcome and the probability of its occurrence. Both have to be seen together, though often the focus is exclusively on outcome, while probability is ignored. The reason for this can be attributed to the generally low probabilities involved. People have cognitive problems in understanding low probabilities, due to a general lack of training in probability theory. For example, try to explain the difference between a probability of 0.01% and 0.001%. Furthermore, often the (unwanted) outcomes cannot be clearly identified. This frequently results in highly uncomfortable situations, both for patients and health care professionals. What is the right course of action?

Let's take a closer look at the two ingredients of risk: undesirable outcomes and uncertainty. Outcomes can be known or unknown; for example, you know that the undesirable outcome of smoking can be lung cancer. On the other hand, in the case of new diseases (such as AIDS in the early 1980s), you may not know what the possible outcomes are.

Similarly, uncertainty can be classified as *aleatory* and *epistemic*. Aleatory uncertainty is the result of a known random process, meaning that you have a fairly good knowledge of the underlying probability distribution. This enables you to state, for instance, that the probability of the unwanted outcome follows a normal distribution. It also permits us to analyse the decision problem at a fairly detailed quantitative level. In the case of epistemic uncertainty, you are faced with a lack of knowledge. You don't know much about the probability distribution and thus it is difficult to perform a valid analysis of the situation.

Given these two dimensions of probability and outcome, you can distinguish between four cases, shown in the risk classification matrix (Figure 11.1). Depending on where you are located in the risk classification matrix, the risk analysis can be

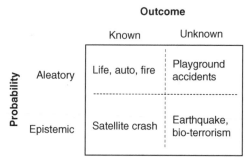

Figure 11.1 The risk classification matrix
Source: Kunreuther (2002)

more or less challenging and call for different tools. In the case of a well-known aleatory risk, with known outcomes, you can use tools such as decision analysis to do a detailed evaluation of the decision problem at hand. For problems in other cells of the risk classification matrix, the analysis will generally be more complex and involve other analysis tools (Paté-Cornell and Murphy, 1996).

Risk management can be thought of as going through five steps: identification, analysis, evaluation of actions, implementations and documentation, as seen in Table 11.1. The first step in risk management is eliciting probable risks. If you were a health official in Toronto in 2003, when China was suffering the first cases of SARS, and you envisioned that some infected patients could travel from China to Toronto, you would have already completed the first important step in managing the corresponding risk and could proceed to Step 2, namely, analysing impact and probability.

Table 11.1 The five steps of risk management

1 Risk identification – determining the possible risks faced by a population, company, etc.
2 Risk analysis – determining the importance of the risk, in terms of probability of occurrence and impact, as well as the expected effect of some alternative actions
3 Action evaluation – determining what can be done to reduce the probability of the event or to mitigate its impact
4 Implementation – ensuring that responsibility for implementing the decided actions is assigned and the decisions are executed
5 Documentation – of the analysis performed, the actions taken and the outcomes. This will allow taking better decisions in the future

Source: Kunreuther (2002)

 Activity 11.1

To illustrate the concept of an – albeit rudimentary – risk analysis, let us assume the following situation: a new disease has struck a city with one million inhabitants. Six hundred individuals have been infected. You can adopt emergency programme A, which will save 200 people with certainty – or, you can adopt emergency programme B, employing a new drug. In this case, there is a probability of 1/3 that all people will be saved and a probability of 2/3 that all will die. What should you do?

 Feedback

Based on this information, you might have drawn a decision tree (Figure 11.2). The rectangle represents the decision, while the circle represents a chance node. The logical flow is from left to right; that is, you first have to decide what to do (choose programme A or programme B), then the uncertainty will be revealed (i.e. if you choose programme B with a probability of 1/3, all 600 people will be saved). This diagram is a clear and concise summary of the decision problem at hand. It does not contain any value judgement, such as 'it would be preferable to avoid the risk of losing all 600 people and thus programme A should be implemented'.

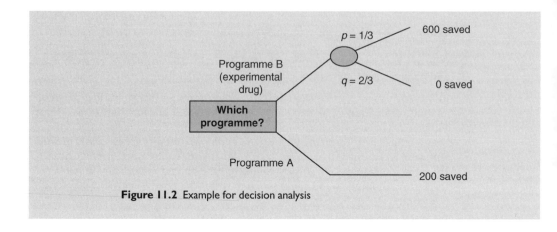

Figure 11.2 Example for decision analysis

When analysing risk, you have to make a clear distinction between good decisions and good outcomes. Unfortunately, the public often confounds the two, particularly in the area of public health. In the example above, a bad decision would be the choice of implementing programme A or programme B *without* previous analysis. A good decision would require a detailed analysis, followed by a value judgement and a choice of programme A or programme B. In the presence of uncertainty, the *outcome* of your decision cannot be influenced by you – that is, your decision to implement programme B does not change the probability of $p = 1/3$ of saving 600 people. But due to our previous analysis, you are able to make an *informed* decision, and thus a good decision.

You also have to clearly distinguish between the risk analysis (which can be made by anybody with experience in the field) and the value judgement, which is reserved for the decision maker (e.g. patient, doctor, health official), based on the previous analysis and her set of preferences. It is very important to realize that different people have different risk profiles. That is, the same risk doesn't mean the same thing to different people; some are more risk-averse, others risk-prone. For example, participating in an experimental drug trial will not be acceptable to a healthy person, while patients with the particular illness to be treated by that drug might exhibit a different preference profile. A curious phenomenon is often present: individuals are risk-seeking when choosing between two losing options but risk-averse when choosing between winning options.

The example shown in Figure 11.2 is a case in point. After having done a detailed risk analysis of the decision problem, the decision analyst and decision maker have come up with the decision tree shown. The analysis of the problem reveals that from the perspective of pure probability theory, alternatives A and B are equivalent in their expected outcomes, as both have an expected value of people saved equal to 200. This addresses the second point, the value judgement. The risk analysis should never be accepted at face value, it needs to be followed by the decision maker's value judgement.

Another important element of the risk assessment health officials must be aware of is how the risk and the situation are being perceived by the public. There is ample scientific evidence that usually the mapping between actual risks and perceived risks is not congruent. This is primarily due to the cognitive inefficiencies of individuals and people's inability to judge (small) probabilities. Furthermore, a number of psychological effects are involved, leading to misperceptions of risk. Among them, you can list voluntary vs. coerced (e.g. working in a nuclear plant vs. living in a nearby village), natural vs. industrial (e.g. sun radiation vs. telephone antennas), familiar vs. not familiar (car driving vs. canoeing), not dreaded vs. dreaded (high blood pressure vs. cancer), chronic vs. catastrophic (car accidents vs. airplane accidents), fair vs. unfair (riding a motorcycle at high speed vs. a pedestrian being hit by the same motorcycle), and so on. Perceived risk is also influenced by imaginability and memorability of hazard (terrorist threats).

Since the late 1970s, a number of publications in scientific journals have dealt with the topic of risk perception. Slovic *et al.* (1979) give comprehensive accounts of a series of studies. Based on the evidence presented, the authors drew the conclusion that there are statistically significant differences in the judgements of risk between experts and lay persons, while expert judgements are closer to the truth than those of the public. Additionally, they noted significant differences between perceived risks and actual risks, as can be seen in Figure 11.3. Here the public's estimates for causes of death are heavily influenced by current issues and less by rational thought.

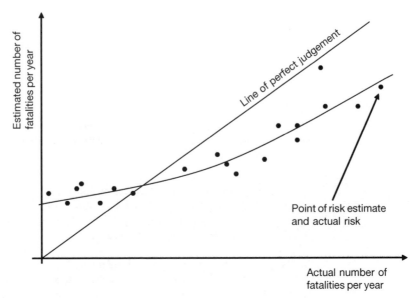

Figure 11.3 Risk perception of the public
Source: Slovic *et al.* (1979)

Research also showed that risks are put into a different order by different groups (e.g. students vs. experts). Perhaps more disturbing is the fact that disagreements about risks cannot be expected to evaporate in the presence of evidence (which often cannot be obtained). This different judgement of risk further complicates the efforts of health policy makers and professionals. Some guidance has been developed by the World Health Organization (Paté-Cornell, 1996).

Once a risk has been analysed, you can move to Step 3, defining risk mitigation measures: to lower the probability of unwanted outcomes or decrease their magnitude. Risk mitigation generally uses two levers: technology and organization. Technology permits you to lower the probability of unwanted outcomes or reduce the severity of unwanted outcomes. Changing standard procedures in the organization allows you to reduce the probability of unwanted outcomes that result from systemic errors in the organization or reduce the negative impact of the unwanted outcome (Paté-Cornell, 1996). Disaster medical services developed in several nations are an example of organizational efforts to lessen the effect of unwanted outcomes (e.g. earthquake, flu epidemic) – much attention has been given to this during the past few years.

The Harvard Medical Practice Study concluded that 'Most medical errors are due to system errors and organizational deficits' (Leape *et al.*, 1991). This emphasizes the importance of organizational awareness in risk mitigation. Unlike the technical side, organizational mitigation often comes at a lower cost (but may encounter resistance from within the organization) and should therefore always be an option to be considered. Here, the health care sector has still a lot to learn from other sectors.

Now having determined what to do, you can progress to Step 4, which consists of implementing the activities, assigning responsibilities in the implementation and ensuring supervision of its evolution. Finally, Step 5 creates and maintains the proper documentation about the decision process, the assumptions made, and the outcomes achieved, and provides the primary source for learning and improving.

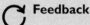 **Activity 11.2**

Consider a normal task that you perform often, like going from home to the video store to rent a movie. You want to watch a particular movie. Go through the first three stages of risk management. In particular:

1 Describe in detail what you plan to do to get the movie – that is, describe the different tasks, who will do them, how long do you expect them to take, etc.
2 Identify the risks that exist in your previous plan. Try to imagine everything that could go wrong with the plan, everything that could prevent you from watching the movie tonight (focus on getting the videotape). Make a list of the risks you encountered.
3 Evaluate the risks, by stating for each one of them its seriousness (i.e. how destructive it can be in terms of your achieving your objective) and its likelihood (i.e. how likely it is for the risk to happen). Now concentrate on the few important risks, in terms of seriousness and/or likelihood.
4 For each of the identified risks, find possible actions that would either mitigate the impact or reduce the probability.

Feedback

To illustrate one possible line of thought, here is a concise answer:

1 To obtain the videotape you plan to drive your car to the video store located on Main Street, rent it and return home. You expect the total time to do it will be around half an hour. You would do this in the late afternoon, just before returning home.

2 The possible risk list may include the following: (1) the car has been stolen, (2) the engine does not start, (3) the store is closed, (4) the store does not carry that movie, (5) the videotape is damaged, etc.

3 You can evaluate the identified risks along the impact and likelihood dimensions, as shown in Figure 11.4

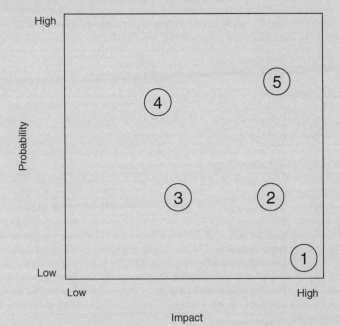

Figure 11.4 Impact and likelihood evaluation

4 For the most important risks, such as the videotape is damaged, you can now plan some actions: check the quality of the videotape in the store, schedule some time in the afternoon to check the quality of the tape, rent a second tape, etc.

Risk communication

Besides risk assessment and development of control actions as described above, there is another area in risk management that becomes critical when a crisis has already occurred involving numerous stakeholders: communicating risk to them. Risk communication is very different from risk analysis in the sense that the public tend to focus on outrage and pay less attention to hazard.

You will learn about two important issues related to risk communication: the dilemmas involved in any communication decision and the use of message maps to convey the desired information to stakeholders.

Communication dilemmas

When organizations face a crisis with a high degree of uncertainty, communication is difficult because how the situation may evolve and how the public will react to the messages are unknown. In this uncertainty, it is hard to decide what information to reveal or to withhold, whether to speculate or not, and so on. Every crisis is different but at the same time many crises are similar, and one of the similarities is that all crises pose pretty much the same dilemmas of communication policy. Crisis experts suggest that institutions should prepare for generic crises before they happen (Mitroff and Anagnos, 2000). These generic crises may include: economic (the sudden collapse of a currency), physical (destruction of a piece of equipment), those related to psychopathic behaviour (product alteration in the market), natural (earthquake), and so on.

Sandman (2002) lists ten communication dilemmas that managers must deal with when addressing communication with the general public and other stakeholders (Table 11.2). Each dilemma can be considered in a continuum from candour, where you may decide to provide as much information as possible, to secrecy, where you may decide to hide as much information as possible (Figure 11.5). Both extremes

Table 11.2 Dilemmas in risk communication

Dilemma extremes	
Candour	Secrecy
Speculation	Refusal to speculate
Tentativeness	Confidence
Being alarming	Being reassuring
Being human	Being professional
Being apologetic	Being defensive
Decentralization	Centralization
Democracy and individual control	Expert decision making
Planning for denial and misery	Planning for panic
Erring on the side of caution	Taking chances

Source: Sandman (2002)

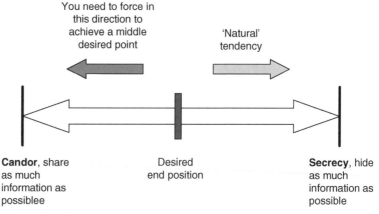

Figure 11.5 The dilemma continuum

Source: Scheme developed by Jaume Ribera based on Sandman (2002)

have clear advantages. In favour of candour would be that people are at their best when collectively facing a difficult situation. The worst is when they find out that they have been misled – then things can get much more unstable, they are more likely to ignore instructions, develop paranoid hypotheses, etc. On the other hand, secrecy might be indicated if the information has not yet been checked. The fear is that people will misunderstand the right information or might panic if they know the whole truth. Another reason would be if opponents take advantage of what is said.

Probably the optimal approach is to strike a balance, providing enough information for the communication receiver to be able to act in a positive way, while not disclosing information that is not sufficiently checked and which could mislead the public. However, in all these dilemmas, you may have a natural tendency towards the right, so, if you wish to end up in a more moderate situation, you will probably have to pull towards the left. Becoming aware of these dilemmas is the first step towards handling them better.

 Activity 11.3

Imagine yourself in a crisis communication situation. You have been left in charge of babysitting your 5-year-old nephew, Andy. He was playing in the park under your supervision. Your phone rings and your sister, Andy's mother, is calling. You look at where your nephew was ten seconds ago and he is no longer there. Your quick visual scan cannot locate him.

Refer to Table 11.2 and identify the corresponding communication dilemmas in your situation. What would the 'average' babysitter do?

 Feedback

As an indication of how to approach the dilemmas, consider the first one: candour versus secrecy. On one extreme, you would tell your sister that you just lost sight of your nephew; on the other extreme, you would assure her that you can see Andy playing and he seems to enjoy it. In favour of the first position is that it would be better that your sister comes if you are really facing a difficult situation. On the other side, the information is not good enough, you have not yet looked around the trees, very likely Andy is playing hide and seek with the other children in the park and your sister might panic unnecessarily.

Message mapping

When a crisis appears, public perceptions and opinions may have as important a role in determining its resolution as executive actions do. If people do not understand the messages directed to them, they will feel irritated and will not follow further advice. On some occasions, people are outraged because they do not understand the risk, and educating the public may work, but in other cases, they do understand the risk and the irritation may be caused by the form of communication (e.g. feeling that the person in charge is withholding information, or receiving what they understand as contradictory versions from different people).

Message mapping is an important tool to assist crisis communication. It aims at achieving message clarity and conciseness and is based on developing a consensus message platform, providing visual aids and road maps for displaying structurally organized responses to anticipated high concern issues, focused at specific stakeholder groups. These are based on widely used mind mapping tools and can be developed manually, or with computer support.

Covello (2002) proposes the following goals of message maps:

- identifying stakeholders early in the communication process
- anticipating stakeholder questions and concerns before they are raised
- organizing thinking and developing prepared messages in response to anticipated stakeholder questions and concerns
- developing key messages and supporting information within a clear, concise, transparent and accessible framework
- promoting open dialogue about messages both inside and outside the organization
- providing user-friendly guidance to spokespersons
- ensuring that the organization has a central repository of consistent messages
- encouraging the organization to speak with one voice

In any crisis it is very helpful to have message maps available (Figure 11.6), both because of the fact of having them and because of the learning and consensus building involved in producing them. A message map will be developed for a specific stakeholder group and for each main concern that affects this group. Therefore, the first stage in developing message maps involves the identification of stakeholder groups and eliciting or discovering their main concerns.

This process can be done in two directions, from the stakeholders to the concerns and vice versa. Some groups prefer a structured 'top-down' approach, first creating a list of stakeholders and then identifying the concerns that they might have. Other groups prefer a 'bottom-up' approach, focusing first on the concerns brought up by the crisis and then identifying which stakeholders may be affected by them. In both cases, what you obtain is a rather extensive list of specific stakeholders and specific concerns that need to be clustered around stakeholder groups and general concerns, in order to bring the list down to a manageable size. Possible stakeholders in a public health case may include the victims and their families, media, emergency response personnel, law enforcement agencies, hospitals and primary health centres and medical associations. The concerns of each group can be drawn from media reports, web pages of activist groups, meeting records, interviews with group representatives, reviews of complaints received, surveys and focus group meetings.

In the second stage, for each of the main stakeholders and their important concerns, you will need to develop the key messages. You can now concentrate on what they most need to know, what they most want to know and what they are most concerned with. Key messages are generally developed in brainstorming sessions with technical experts, communication specialists, legal advisors and possibly a facilitator. The objective of this phase is to create a set of key messages, addressing a concern of a stakeholder group. A key message may consist of a whole

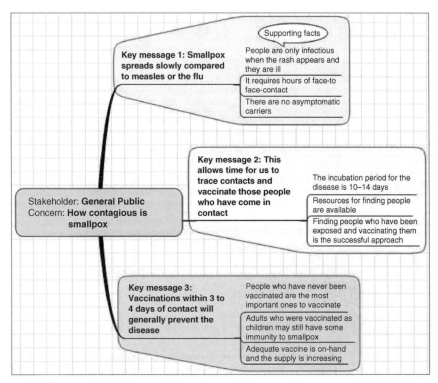

Figure 11.6 Message map of the general public's concern about smallpox
Source: Covello (2002)

sentence or just two or three keywords, which will later be developed into full messages.

It is worth noting that when people are upset and under stress they may suffer what is known as 'mental noise', the inability to hear, understand and remember what is being conveyed to them. In these cases, it is important to limit the number of key messages to three and keep them brief, clear and concise. When possible, include the key concepts at the beginning and/or at the end of the message, and if time allows use the three-T approach: tell the audience what you are about to tell them, tell them and, finally, tell them what you have told them.

In the third stage, you will need to develop supporting facts and arguments as proof of the messages. Even though you will probably not include these in the primary message, they may be very handy if a particular message is challenged by someone in the audience. As a final stage, before the message is delivered, it is prudent to conduct some testing, presenting the messages to experts and surrogate target audiences, both internal and external.

For Activities 11.4 and 11.5, choose either Version a or b for both. Answer the questions yourself first and then invite friends and family to answer the same questions. Compare the answers you obtain.

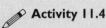 **Activity 11.4**

Imagine that your government is preparing for the outbreak of an unusual disease which is expected to kill 600 people. Two alternative programmes to combat the disease have been proposed. Assume that the exact scientific estimate of the consequences of the programmes are as follows:

(a) If programme A is adopted, 200 people will be saved.
(b) If programme B is adopted, there is a 1/3 probability that 600 people will be saved, and a 2/3 probability that no people will be saved

Which programme would you choose?

Feedback

This gives an example of the *framing effect* in decision making (Tversky and Kahneman, 1982).

An analysis from a risk-neutral perspective shows that in each group, the 'sure bet' and 'gamble' alternatives have the same expected outcome: 200 survivors. Calculation: you have to choose between (i) '200 people will be saved' and (ii) 1/3 probability of saving all and a 2/3 probability of no survivors. The calculation for (ii) (risk-neutral decision maker) would be 1/3*600 survivors + 2/3 *0 survivors = 200 survivors – that is, the same expected value as in (i) (the same applies for group b). From this perspective, there is no difference between formulation a and formulation b of the decision problem of exercise 1. So what is different?

In the first example, the decision problem is framed in a positive way ('will be saved'). Generally, option (a) '200 people will be saved' is preferred. This is an example of risk-averse behaviour (i.e. avoid risks). In the second example, the decision problem is framed in a negative way ('will die'). Generally, option (b) '2/3 probability that 600 will die' is preferred. This is risk-prone behaviour (i.e. gambling).

 Activity 11.5

You have been exposed to a rare fatal disease and now face a chance of 0.001 of quick and painless death within two weeks. What percentage of the total amount you expect to earn during your lifetime would you be willing to pay to reduce this probability to 0 (e.g. by buying a new medicine)?

Now assume that:

(a) If programme A is adopted, 400 people will die.
(b) If programme B is adopted, there is a 1/3 probability that nobody will die, and a 2/3 probability that 600 people will die.

Which programme would you choose?

Now consider that you have been asked to participate in a medical experiment involving a new drug that will cure a deadly disease. There is a chance of 0.001 of quick and painless death in the course of this experiment. What percentage of your expected life net income would make you willing to participate in this experiment (e.g. by buying a new medicine)?

Feedback

This gives an example of the loss aversion and voluntary vs. involuntary risks. People are more sensitive to the dimension in which they are losing relative to their reference point. There is a great difference between willingness-to-accept (WTA) and willingness-to-pay (WTP) in situations with voluntary assumption of additional risk – and situations of failure to reduce or eliminate existing risk.

In the first example, the problem was framed as one of being ill and looking for a cure, while in the second example subjects can voluntarily expose themselves to a risk of the given magnitude. Answers will differ significantly, while from a risk-neutral perspective they should be identical.

Activity 11.6

Scientific evidence suggests that disease X occurs with a frequency of one-in-a-thousand in cattle. Government agencies have funded extensive research into animal testing and a pharmaceutical company has recently developed a new test that is more reliable at identifying cattle with disease X. Results show that the probability of a true positive (i.e. if the test indicates that an animal is infected, it is) is 99%, while the probability of a true negative (i.e. the test says that the animal is not infected and it isn't) is 98%.

When the Minister of Agriculture presents the new test to the public on national news, the results for a cow are shown and the test says that it is infected.

What is the probability that the cow is infected? >60% or <60%?

Feedback

The correct answer is significantly smaller than 60%, which may surprise you.

Summary

You have seen how risk assessment is the process by which risks are identified and quantified and risk management is the process by which this information is used in making decisions to reduce or eliminate the risk. When there are fundamental uncertainties in a problem, there is often a tendency to resort to 'conservative estimates' – which then add up to a model that is far too conservative. Risk management in the public sector must address: economic efficiency and justice and equity. You have learnt how there is a lack of consistency in public decision making in the face of risk. An essential ingredient in any risk management programme is that of risk communication. When addressing a crisis, health officials should not only consider the critical elements of risk (probability and impact) but also the outrage experienced by the population. Message mapping is an effective way to identify stakeholders early in the communication process, anticipate their questions and concerns before they are raised, and prepare key messages and supporting information within a clear, concise, transparent and accessible framework. It is also a great tool to open an internal dialogue among the professionals and to develop consensus on how to handle typical communication dilemmas.

References

Committee on Risk Perception and Communication (1989) *Improving Risk Communication.* Washington, DC: National Academy Press

Covello V (2002) *Message Mapping.* WHO Workshop on Bioterrorism. Geneva: WHO

Kunreuther H (2002) Risk analysis and risk management in an uncertain world, *Risk Analysis* 22(4): 655–64

Leape LL, Brennan TA, Laird N, Lawthers AG, Localio AR, Barnes BA *et al.* (1991) The nature of adverse events in hospitalized patients: results of the Harvard Medical Practice Study II. *New England Journal of Medicine* 324(6): 377–84

Mitroff II, Anagnos G (2000) *Managing Crises Before They Happen: What Every Executive and Manager Needs to Know About Crisis Management.* New York: Amacom

Paté-Cornell ME (1996) Uncertainties in risk analysis: six levels of treatment, *Reliability Engineering and Systems Safety* 54: 95–111

Paté-Cornell ME, Murphy DM (1996) Human and management factors in probabilistic risk analysis: the SAM approach and observations from recent applications, *Reliability Engineering and Systems Safety* 53: 115–26

Sandman PM (2002) *Dilemmas in Emergency Communication Policy. Emergency Risk Communication CDCynergy.* Atlanta, GA: Centers for Disease Control and Prevention, US Department of Health and Human Services (CD-ROM)

Slovic P, Fischoff B, Lichenstein S (1979) Rating the risks, *Environment* 2: 14–20

Tversky A, Kahneman D (1982) Judgment under uncertainty: heuristics and biases, in Kahneman D, Slovic P, Tversky A (eds.) *Judgment Under Uncertainty: Heuristics and Biases.* Cambridge: Cambridge University Press.

Further reading

Bennett P, Calman K (1999). Risk Communication and Public Health. Oxford: Oxford University Press

12

Application of models of behaviour change

Overview

In this chapter, you will consider the application of models of behaviour change as they apply to the promotion of health and the prevention of disease. You will learn about their principal strengths and weaknesses, see how to place these models and their implications within a societal framework, and learn how best to use the models in practice, in meaningful and useful ways.

Learning objectives

By the end of the chapter, you will be able to:

- understand the idea of applying models of behaviour change to appropriate situations in health promotion
- describe the strengths and weaknesses associated with modelling behaviour change
- consider the relationship between describing behaviour change using models and bringing about change on health behaviour in practice
- analyse a health promotion scenario involving health-related behaviour change

Key terms

Models of behaviour change Representations of how people think and act and the ways in which this can be changed; used to help predict and explain behaviour.

Introduction

It is often suggested that changing people's behaviour is at the heart of health promotion. The reason for this is that in high-income countries, the pattern of disease and illness is partly determined by people's behaviour. Cancer and heart disease, which account for most premature mortality, have aetiologies to which behaviour contributes. Activities such as smoking, overeating fatty foods, not consuming enough fresh fruit and vegetables and not taking enough exercise, all contribute to the risk of heart disease and cancer. Sexually transmitted infections, liver disease and children's immunological status are also affected by people's choices about their behaviour, their alcohol consumption and whether they get their children immunized. These things are, theoretically at least, within the realms of individual choice and responsibility. It also follows therefore that because human behaviour plays such a role, a dividend of prevention is within grasp, if people were to change their behaviour (Kelly and Capewell, 2004; Kelly *et al.*, 2004a). Of course, human behaviour and therefore behaviour change are actually only part of the story and the wider determinants of health are vitally important.

This chapter emphasizes the social context of individual behaviour change and the practical steps and considerations health promoters need to consider to support behaviour change in ways that are empathetic and consequently more likely to be effective.

In this context, health promotion interventions tend to focus on preventing or reducing risky behaviours such as unsafe sex, poor eating habits and smoking, or by promoting health protective behaviours such as screening, immunization and taking exercise. Interventions may attempt to do this by, for example, increasing knowledge and awareness of services to help to prevent risk. Interventions may also seek to change attitudes, for example by communicating messages about the harm that smoking does to the lungs and cardiovascular system. Another approach is to increase physical or interpersonal skills, for example on how to use condoms or how to use assertiveness skills in sexual encounters. Some interventions are designed to change beliefs and perceptions, such as those aimed at increasing testicular self-examination in men by raising their awareness of risk and normalizing self-examination. Another approach is to influence social norms, for example about public perceptions of the harm of second-hand smoke inhalation or public acceptance of breast feeding.

Models of behaviour change

There is a considerable amount of research about changing people's beliefs and attitudes about health and about changing health-damaging or promoting health-enhancing behaviours (Anderson, 1988; Kaplan *et al.*, 1993). A great deal of this research involves the use of models. As you learnt in Chapter 3, a model is a schematic representation and simplification of some complex process.

There are a number of general points to make at the outset about models of behaviour change and their use in practice. Models tend to operate at fairly high levels of generality. This obviously aids simplification and understanding. On the other hand, it can make applying them to real-world situations a little tricky because real life tends to be complex and messy. As you saw earlier, models that are multi-level – that is, which operate at the individual *and* social level and which take into account the needs and the characteristics of particular population groups – work best. Unfortunately, the more particular the local characteristics and needs of the population, the more complex the models become and the advantages of simplicity can get lost. So in practical terms in real-life interventions, practitioners change and amend models to suit their needs. While this of course is an entirely sensible thing to do from a practical point of view, it often means that the models do not appear to work very well from a scientific point of view. No single model or theory has been shown to be universally applicable, although many can accurately predict and describe some changes, particularly when they are focused on individual level factors.

There is a large amount of research dealing with these matters. It originally developed in the late 1940s in the USA when the first effective vaccines against poliomyelitis were developed. In spite of the availability of an effective vaccine, the uptake was relatively low. In fact, there was an epidemic of cases in the USA after the development and availability of the vaccine. Two questions emerged from this. What were the factors which led to this type of behaviour despite the availability of information? And, what could be done to change it? Models that have been designed to answer these questions have since been applied to all sorts of health behaviour such as the use of contraception, smoking cessation, oral health, taking exercise and alcohol misuse (see Kaplan *et al.*, 1993).

 Activity 12.1

Think back to Chapter 3, in which you were introduced to three theories that help to explain health behaviour and health behaviour change at an individual level (the health belief model, the stages of change or transtheoretical model, and social cognitive theory). What are the main features of these models?

 Feedback

The health belief model illustrates the importance of individual beliefs about health and the costs and benefits of actions to protect and improve health. It suggests that the likelihood of a person taking action is based on the interaction between four types of belief related to the condition or problem: perceived susceptibility; perceived seriousness; availability of a course of action that will reduce susceptibility; and the perceived benefits and barriers to action.

The stages of change model is based on the premise that behaviour change is a *process*. Five basic stages of change are identified: pre-contemplation, contemplation, determination (or preparation), action and maintenance. The model suggests that it is important to understand what stage a person is at and develop strategies appropriate for that stage.

Social cognitive theory highlights the importance of the interaction between an individual and their environment.

Taken together, the models emphasize:

- the importance of knowledge and beliefs about health
- the importance of self-efficacy: the belief in one's competency to take action
- the importance of perceived social norms and social influences related to the value an individual places on social approval or acceptance by different social groups
- the importance of recognizing that individuals in a population may be at different stages of change at any one time

- limitations to psycho-social theories which do not adequately take account of socio-economic and environmental conditions that significantly shape access to services and resources
- the importance of shaping or changing the environment or people's perception of the environment as an important element of programmes.

Effectiveness of models

Recent reviews of the effectiveness of interventions have found that interventions using a theory-based approach – regardless of what theory they used – tended to be more effective than those that did not, indicating perhaps that using a theory-based approach to plan interventions may make an intervention better planned and delivered. Models provide the basis for increased rigour in intervention design. Model-based interventions are necessarily more explicit. Exner *et al.* (1997) identify an important design component as 'having explicitly stated goals or hypotheses, with clearly operationalized outcomes'. Models require that the intervention articulates the determinants that influence behavioural and clinical outcomes and are explicit about which of these they propose to change; how they propose to change them; how they will demonstrate that change; and how, if at all, that change has contributed to a behavioural or clinical outcome.

Models also help you to know why, as well as whether, an intervention is effective, shedding light on the extent to which elements of interventions can be applied in different contexts with different populations. Different models work better in relation to some conditions or preventive actions rather than others. Approaches that can accommodate irrational behaviour and incorporate the function of wider determinants tend to cover a broader range of potential issues but to be less good when dealing with specifics and guiding interventions.

No single theory or model has universal applicability and the choice of a particular approach should depend on what the focus for change is. No single theory or model can universally predict behavioural intentions or outcomes for all populations, although many can accurately predict and describe some changes, particularly when they are focused on the individual. They tend to be less good at incorporating structural or socio-economic factors.

There are two limitations associated with these types of models: empirical and theoretical-ontological. The empirical problem is that where the models are used there is sometimes considerable variance in their predictive power. Unfortunately, it is unclear whether this is caused by poor design and method or underlying weakness in the models. Another problem is the propensity for practitioners to change components of the model to suit their needs. The reason for this is the need to ground the models in the real world and to operationalize the components in them to suit local circumstances. It is also very important to acknowledge that notions like attitude, intention, belief and assessment of risk are much easier to talk about in the abstract than to apply to real settings and to real people.

The theoretical-ontological problem is more serious. This is about the explanatory focus on the individual to the exclusion of the social in these models and many like them. Where social factors are included in these models, they are invariably treated as characteristics of individuals and hence as part of an individually driven explanation, rather than explanatory causes in their own right. Consequently, social structure is not dealt with adequately. It is treated as a set of individually expressed factors, not as a highly variegated pattern of social arrangements requiring their own level of analysis, irreducible to the individual. The population is not homogeneous. It is heterogeneous and its component parts respond to the same interventions in different ways. However, these models generally assume universal precepts about human behaviour or treat social differences as confounding factors in the analysis. In other words, the key differences between social classes, men and women, ethnic groups, young and old, and residential circumstances are treated as background or contextual factors, rather than important determining factors in their own right. Different segments of the population respond in very different ways to the same intervention by virtue of their social differences and attempting to apply general principles across the whole population tend to under-emphasize the important role of social difference (Killoran and Kelly, 2004).

In spite of the general problems attaching to these approaches, it is important to remember that from a practical point of view, the logical imperfections and the scientific limitations of the models are much less important than their ability to help us to bring about change in real time for real people. These models point us in the right direction and provide us with a framework for thinking about interventions. If they are treated as a recipe for determining exactly what should be done, in each and every circumstance, they will disappoint. If they are treated as signposts for action, they can be very helpful indeed (Kelly *et al.*, 2004b).

 Activity 12.2

Write down some examples of models of human behaviour change drawn from your own experience. These need not necessarily be from the field of health promotion. What sorts and ranges of behaviour are health promoters aiming to change to improve health? Think about all the different sorts of people and organizations that are interested in behaviour change, including schools, prisons, retailers and governments. Draw on your understanding of the range of impacts health promotion aims to have on different sectors and different communities, as well as individuals.

 Feedback

There are no right answers here but your list should have included not just individual behaviours, such as smoking and eating, but actions such as enabling access to healthy foods through changing the behaviour of food producers and retailers. Improving educational attainments through changes in truancy and school absences might be another area of behaviour change you thought of.

Practical steps to interventions

The right direction indicated in the models needs to be given some practical substance. There are a number of aspects to this.

Choice of theory or model

The choice of theory or model to guide the intervention should be made on the basis of the problem being tackled. Multi-level approaches can be delivered by different mechanisms, so you need to think about mechanisms and media. For example, information from mass media campaigns can reach a large proportion of the population very quickly (although such campaigns may miss the very poor). Tailored health information delivered via health professionals or others who work one to one with people, will take longer to filter through but may produce a stronger response because of its tailored and direct nature. Using mass media and professionals together may be highly synergistic and work better so long as it is integrated. A good example of such an integrated approach is the 'back to sleep' campaign which began in 1991 following an expert group report that young babies should be placed on their backs to sleep to help to prevent sudden infant death syndrome. The campaign included mass media and health professionals delivering individually targeted information and advice. The rate of cot death in many European countries fell significantly.

Recognition of context

Local circumstances and the engagement of local practitioners have a considerable effect on the success or otherwise of an intervention. So consideration must be given to the ways that the professionals who are to deliver it might respond. However, the prime basis for any intervention should be the group or population who are the focus of attention. An assessment of their needs and characteristics is the platform on which everything else rests. It is therefore particularly important to develop an understanding of what the world feels like when viewed from the perspective of these people. It is important for the health professional *not* to assume that they know what the needs and characteristics of their target group are in advance. One of the most important things to do at this point is to try to discard prejudices and stereotypes of the type 'all white middle-class people are so and so, all Afro-Caribbean men are such and such, and men who have sex with men are thus and thus', and so on. It is of course never possible to know the way others truly think and feel, but it is important to try to get close to it.

There are numerous ways of ascertaining such information, but in practical terms talking and listening is as good a place to start as any. It is not a good idea to propose a large research project to find these things out. This will be slow and time-consuming. Enough can be gleaned by listening and learning, both from the people themselves and from the professionals who work with them. What does the target group know and understand about the issue you as a health promoter want to work with them on? What do they think and feel about it? What do they think they need to know about it? Do they see it as a problem for them and for others? Also, do they have any sense of where you are coming from as a health promoter? Focus group activity is usually the best way to draw out such knowledge and understanding quickly. The point is to try to see the world from the position of those whose behaviour you wish to influence or to change.

One very important element in this is to try to find out as much as possible about the benefits and disbenefits of the proposed change in behaviour viewed from the position of the target group. For example, smoking and drinking alcohol clearly provide very supportive and integral parts of people's lives. People who do heavy manual labour may consume large quantities of beer as a means of replacing fluid, and a cigarette break has been a traditional and tolerated way of taking a short break from physical labour in many jobs involving hard effort. Smoking also performs a valuable function for many by providing a pleasant feeling of mild intoxication and a shot of relief at times of stress or trouble, or to help relax. To lose sight of these important dimensions of people's lives is to misunderstand the very people you seek to help. To view the smoking habits of manual workers or single mothers in straitened economic circumstances from the perspective of the risk adverse middle classes is a misjudgement on a par with colonialists' ignorance of the lifestyles of their subjects. When conducting campaigns designed to change people we must take care not to invent some new, more insidious form of internal colonialism. You must try to know and to understand the world of the people you seek to help.

The next element is to consider the kinds of skills you need to equip people with to help them change. There are broadly speaking four kinds of skills: technical, interpersonal, intrapersonal and inter-subjective.

Technical skills

These skills are about the technical hand skills, knowledge and confidence to do the new behaviour. For example, some smokers will need new ways to use their hands in the absence of the paraphernalia of cigarettes, lighters and matches. If you want people to start exercising, you need to help them to understand about proper warming up, how to start, how to pace themselves, how not to put themselves at risk and what clothes will be comfortable (as well as fashionable). If you want to talk about healthy eating, you have to think about healthy shopping, budgeting and cooking. These are considerable skills in their own right. The amount of information and sheer necessity of demonstrating them should not be underestimated. It is vital to remember that simply telling someone how to do something – or telling them that they ought to do something – is, generally speaking, not the best way to impart a skill. Nor, of course, is writing it down and giving it to them in a leaflet. You need to show them how to do it and perhaps back it up with other kinds of materials.

Interpersonal skills

These are about teaching the person how to manage interactions with others as they engage in their new ways of behaving. So the smoker who wants to quit needs to learn how to refuse cigarettes from former fellow smokers who will undoubtedly sometimes try to make themselves feel better by trying to undermine the efforts of someone trying to quit. The giving-up smoker will need to know what to say in order to say 'no'. The person managing a sexual encounter may need to know the interpersonal skills of managing such encounters, and of learning the etiquette of sexual intercourse or refusal to have sex. The busy mother trying to introduce a healthier diet onto the family tea table needs to anticipate the rejection that new menus might evoke from children and partners.

The reason why interpersonal skills are so important is that all human behaviour, including health behaviour, happens in social contexts. Patterns of human behaviour in these social contexts tend to have an habitual quality. Therefore, breaking the habit, which is what much of human behaviour actually is, involves doing things differently. This is sometimes very difficult to do without support. Not surprisingly, it is sometimes far easier to change an habitual behaviour when other things in life change, like changing a job, moving house, having a baby or ending a relationship. These are all really good points in life to make changes in health behaviours because of the loss of some of the things that reinforced the types of behaviour which people may want to change.

Intrapersonal skills

This refers to the emotional and expressive feelings that people experience in any human behaviour and which they attach to human contact and encounters. These have a particular salience in the context of health behaviours and changes to health behaviours. So, there may be feelings of loss attached to the absence of previously valued behaviours and rewards from those behaviours like smoking. People may genuinely miss it and yearn to be like they were before, even though they may recognize the benefits of giving up. The companionship, the intoxication, the sense of doing something with one's hands may all provide the props and parts of the script to everyday life for typical smokers. These things will be missed. There may also be intense feelings of frustration and anger, as the giving-up smoker experiences withdrawal symptoms. There may be similar feelings of loss if people stop eating large amounts of sweet and fatty foods. Chocolate and cakes may become objects of fixation or of loss. Using condoms may lead to feelings of lack of intimacy in sexual relationships. At a more general level, the whole approach to leading a healthier life may be seen either as something to be valued or regarded by the people whose behaviour is being changed as an intense interference to individual freedom. You have to help clients both work through and prepare for these feelings in advance. It is very important not to underestimate the intensity of feelings, positive and negative, linked to so much of what we might wish to change, and not to undersell these to clients.

Subjective skills

Subjective skills are to do with helping the client make sense of it all. The issues you are dealing with here, the things which are the targets of the health promoter's attempts to change, are central to the ways people live their lives and are integral to their sense of whom and what they think they are. Their sense of self and their sense of identity, indeed the very ways they make sense of the world and their place in the world, are deeply embedded in what they eat, drink, their sex lives, their smoking, and so on. When you ask someone to change, in varying degrees you are asking them to be a different person to the one that they habitually think of themselves as being and to break emotional bonds with significant others in important ways. So deciding to stop smoking is not a simple choice like deciding that you prefer one cheese to another. The decisions you are asking of people are not to make a choice between living a healthy life or an unhealthy one. Rather, you are asking them to take actions that will essentially change the nature of the person that they are. So obviously you must not just dump down in front of them the options to smoke or not to smoke, or to eat a low-fat or a high-fat diet. It is about much more fundamental processes of helping the target population come to terms with the changes they may genuinely want to make, and working through the processes of change. It is about understanding the barriers to change, most of which while structurally determined exist in the micro world, the life world, of the individuals you hope to influence. Those barriers are generated in the mind and everyday interactions of the individuals themselves, as well as the social structure they inhabit. So at the heart of any attempt to change behaviour, there must be ways of helping the people who you want to do things differently make sense of it. That is why you need to understand the world from their point of view before you start. That is why simply telling someone it is for their own good, or that it is a simple choice, is inadequate.

 Activity 12.3

Imagine you are a health promoter and you have been asked to organize a health promotion intervention in hospital and community settings in your capital city, to increase the number of new mothers who both start and continue to breastfeed for at least nine months. Think first about how you would construct a list of objectives for such an intervention. You may need to look back over the theories of organizational change and planning steps in Chapter 4. Many different aspects of services may need to be involved, and a variety of professionals too. And don't forget the mothers! Then identify some of the specifics of the intervention that might be applied. Consider how much involves behaviour change and how much organizational change. In behavioural terms, what are the key intervention points? Finally, list the practical problems that might be encountered and describe the kinds of solutions you might apply to overcome those problems.

Feedback

Keep the notes of this activity to hand as you move onto the next chapter on health promotion planning, which will look at these stages in more detail.

Summary

You have seen how behaviour change operates at different levels. Organizational features set the context within which decisions are made at the individual level. As the models of behaviour change show, there are complex human calculations in operation as people work through the decision they make. There is a process which the decision-making path follows and there will be a variety of potential cues to action. There is also a range of practical things that can be done which depend on four types of skill – technical, interpersonal, intrapersonal and inter-subjective. These have to be applied with an understanding of the life worlds of those you want to help. The models are your starting point. They provide you with a set of signposts about the direction in which you can go. However, the practical problems that reside within people's everyday life worlds have to be solved, and using the schema here, it is perfectly possible to tease out the critical issues and work them through.

References

Anderson R (1988) The development of the concept of health behaviour and its application to recent research, in Anderson R, Davies JK, Kickbusch I, McQueen DV, Turner J (eds.) *Health Behaviour Research and Health Promotion*. Oxford: Oxford University Press

Azjen I (1985) From intentions to actions: a theory of planned behaviour, in Kuhl J, Beckman J (eds.) *Action Control from Cognition to Behaviour*. New York: Springer-Verlag

Exner TM, Seal DW, Ehrhardt AA (1997) A review of HIV interventions for at-risk women, *AIDS and Behavior* 1(2): 93–124

Fishbein M, Azjen I (1975) *Belief, Attitude, Intention and Behavior: An Introduction to Theory and Research*. Reading, MA: Addison-Wesley

Fisher JD, Fisher WA (2000) Theoretical approaches to individual-level change in HIV risk behaviour, in Peterson JL, DiClemente RJ (eds.) *Handbook of HIV Prevention*. New York: Kluwer Academic/Plenum Publishers

Fisher WA, Fisher JD (1993) A general social psychological model for changing AIDS risk behaviour, in Pryor J, Reeder G (eds.) *The Social Psychology of HIV Infection*. Hillsdale, NJ: Erlbaum.

Kaplan RM, Sallis JF, Patterson TL (1993) *Health and Human Behavior*. New York: McGraw-Hill

Kelly MP, Capewell S (2004) *Relative Contributions of Changes in Risk Factors and Treatment to the Reduction of Coronary Heart Disease Mortality*. London: Health Development Agency

Kelly MP, Crombie H, Owen L (2004a) *The Contribution of Smoking, Diet, Screening and Treatment to Cancer Mortality in the Under 75s*. London: Health Development Agency (available at: http://www.publichealth.nice.org.uk/documents/cancer_under75s_briefing.pdf)

Kelly MP, Speller V, Meyrick J (2004b) *Getting Evidence into Practice in Public Health*. London: Health Development Agency (available at: http://www.publichealth.nice.org.uk/documents/getting_eip_pubhealth.pdf)

Killoran A, Kelly MP (2004) Towards an evidence-based approach to tackling health inequalities: the English experience, *Health Education Journal* 63: 7–14

13

Planning a health promotion intervention

Overview

In this chapter, you will examine the planning process for a health promotion intervention. In previous chapters, you have dealt with specific issues in developing a health promotion programme and have highlighted a range of methodologies available for use. In Chapters 3 and 4, you looked at theories underpinning health promotion and were introduced to some of the models that will be considered in this chapter. In Chapter 14, you will look at the detail of planning evaluation. This chapter presents you with information about areas to think about in planning an intervention from start to finish and provides you with an overview of some of the planning tools currently available that can help you to ensure quality in your intervention. It is a practically oriented chapter that will help you apply your learning about health promotion to the systematic planning of health promotion activities.

Learning objectives

After you have worked through this chapter, you will better be able to:

- understand the basic stages required to plan a health promotion intervention
- methodically plan a health promotion intervention
- draw upon available planning tools to help ensure the creation of a quality health promotion intervention

Key terms

Context The circumstances surrounding an intervention, including cultural environment, political environment, existing work related to the intervention, current events shaping opinion on the topic, etc.

Programme development The design of an intervention with consideration given to identified needs, aims, objectives and contextual factors, such as cultural and political environment.

Programme evaluation Assessment of the value of a programme.

Programme implementation The act of applying a programme taking into account resources and target population.

Sustainability The extent to which an intervention may be continued beyond its initial implementation; this may be dependent upon a continued source of funding, programme effectiveness, or changing priorities.

Target group The group to which an intervention is addressed.

Planning a health promotion intervention

 Activity 13.1

Before you familiarize yourself with the most important stages of health promotion programme planning, consider the key steps you would go through if you were to plan a health promotion intervention. Write down these key steps and brief descriptions of what they might entail. Be sure you are considering complete programme planning, working from programme development through programme evaluation. You may find some guidance by looking at the key terms provided above.

 Feedback

The descriptions below consider the key stages in planning a health promotion intervention. Have you included all of these in your answer? If there are some you have overlooked, take some extra time to read their descriptions and consider their importance for programme planning.

Although there is a range of tools to help you plan an effective health promotion intervention, there is a basic model that will ensure that no key stage is missed. The detail of each stage is dealt with elsewhere in this book but the most important stages are discussed in turn.

Assess need

This may require you to use a range of sources, such as:

- epidemiological data
- demographic and socio-economic information
- the felt need of the target audience
- the perceived need of professionals who work with the target audience
- assets which the target group may possess that you will be able to build upon

From this information you should be able to identify clearly the target group for your intervention, understand the nature of the problem and be aware of any assets currently in existence.

At the assessment stage, you should also consider the political climate and whether your intervention will garner the necessary support from those in key decision-making roles. For instance, will you receive permission to carry out the work from those who need to give it or approval from those who will be required to fund it?

Try to balance those aspects which you think will help your intervention and those that will hinder it. Examples might include the presence of lots of human capital but a lack of access to services, or the availability of funds, but only for the period when weather would limit the ability to work in the target geographical area.

Interrogate the evidence base

Once you have defined the problem, or the assets you wish to enhance, you will need to look to international literature sources to determine what interventions have been shown to work in this situation (which will be discussed in Chapter 15). You may also draw upon learning from similar pieces of work that you know have taken place in a comparable cultural setting but which have not appeared in the literature. Care should be taken to examine the evaluation of any intervention that you intend to emulate, to ensure that you are learning from good practice and will not repeat the mistakes of others.

Identify resources

Resources may be equipment, financial or human. Consider those which will help with the intervention practically on the implementation level and those which will give political support as a resource.

Inevitably, you will have finite resources, so you will need to plan an intervention that is realistically achievable within those confines. However, you may wish to develop a proposal for additional resources. In this case, it is best to leave this stage until the other stages of the plan have been completed.

Aims

Identify what you hope the intervention will achieve. For example, you may be working towards a health improvement or behaviour change. Identifying your aims at the outset will help to orient you during the planning process and will ultimately assist in evaluating the programme.

Targets

Sometimes the most effective way to demonstrate success is by using a numerical target. An example of a numerical target would be: to reduce the rate of smoking in 11–14 year old girls in Riga by 10 per cent by the year 2015. However, to set this type of target, you need accurate baseline data. In this instance, you would need accurate data about the smoking rate at the outset of your intervention. You will also need to take care when designing the evaluation, so that your methodology will produce the right sort of data to demonstrate progress against the target.

Objectives

Objectives are the specific actions you will take to achieve the aim.

Methodology

These are the techniques you will employ to operationalize your objectives to meet your overall aims.

Evaluation

It is important that health promotion interventions are evaluated, not only so that you can be sure that your intervention is achieving the desired outcome, but also to add to the evidence base for health promotion. Chapter 14 will deal with appropriate evaluation methodologies.

Resource allocation and budget setting

If this was not completed earlier, it will be important at this stage to identify what resources will be required for your intervention to be successful. This should include a budget that details the costs over the duration of the intervention. If the budget exceeds what is available, you may need to prioritize areas of your work. Examples might be reducing the number of participants, or omitting one of the inputs. However, it may be that a reduction in funding will compromise the proposed intervention to a point where it is no longer viable. In this case, it is better to accept than to start an intervention that has little chance of success.

Implementation of the intervention should not commence until all of these stages have been adequately addressed.

 Activity 13.2

To understand properly the steps outlined above, it is useful to plan a sample intervention utilizing them. Take some time now to plan a smoking intervention using these key planning stages. When planning your intervention, make certain you are clear about your specific aim; perhaps you are planning a programme to prevent young children from smoking later in life or maybe you wish to design an intervention aimed at helping elderly smokers to quit. Think critically about each stage in the planning process and be very specific with your target group, aims and objectives. Be sure you are considering each step carefully. Record all the information as you will be using it in a later Activity.

Feedback

Go back through your planning process and compare it with the stages listed above. Have you included all of them? You should have assessed need by gathering data about populations at increased need for an intervention. You also should have undertaken a search to determine whether it is reasonable to expect support from community members and leaders for this type of intervention. Have you looked at the evidence base to identify existing smoking interventions? Were you able to determine any potential sources of support for your programme through community or government organizations? If you cannot clearly answer these questions, return to your plan to further elaborate on them.

Re-examine your aims. They should be clearly stated so that an independent evaluator would be able to determine easily whether your programme does indeed achieve what you set out to do. The same is true for your targets. Have a second look at them to determine if they are too broad. If there is no numerical or other clear target for success included, consider rewriting the targets in a more concrete fashion.

Have your objectives been reasonably set? Go back and look at your objectives and methodology to determine if they are feasible in the context of information you have gathered about resources and from the evidence base. Also reconsider whether your objectives will be useful to reach your aims and targets for your specific target group.

Finally, think about your evaluation. This should capture whether you have achieved your aims and reached your targets. Will it do this? Does your evaluation produce the kind of results that could be included in an evidence base? If not, re-work your evaluation so its outcomes are useful pieces of information that can be included in the evidence base or as support for future project funding. This does not mean changing the evaluation so that it provides only data that indicate your intervention was successful, but rather adjusting the terms of evaluation so that it produces information that will show whether you have or have not achieved what you set out to do.

It may be more difficult for you to carry out the final stage of resource allocation and budget setting in an exercise such as this but think about what you would omit if you had budget shortcomings. Consider whether or not your programme would be viable if you encountered a lack of funding.

Planning tools for health promotion

Now that you have planned a programme on your own and have a better understanding of the key stages involved, it will be helpful to know that there are many sophisticated tools that can be employed in the planning process that can help to ensure the quality of the intervention. These tools use a variety of approaches to carry out the stages in planning with which you are now familiar. Inevitably, the process will vary depending upon the type of intervention, the target group, and the size and scope of the intervention. However, it is helpful to have a general tool for use in planning a health promotion programme or intervention to ensure that no key steps are neglected. Several planning tools have been developed. A selection of these, which characterize differing approaches, are highlighted in Table 13.1.

Table 13.1 A selection of planning tools for health promotion

Planning tool	Web address
Programme Management Guidelines for Health Promotion	http://www.commed.unsw.edu.au/cgpis/public/PHCReD/Programme%20Management%20Guidelines.pdf
The Public Health Bush Book, Vol. I	http://www.nt.gov.au/health/healthdev/health_promotion/bushbook/bushbook_toc.shtml
Preffi-Health Promotion Effect Management Instrument	http://w3.nigz.nl/docfiles/Explanatory_Guide.PDF, http://w3.nigz.nl/docfiles/Assesment_package_Preffi_211.pdf
PRECEDE-PROCEED	http://lgreen.net/precede.htm; http://www.med.usf.edu/~kmbrown/PRECEDE_PROCEED_Overview.htm, http://www.ulm.edu/education/hhp/PRECEDE-PROCEED.html, http://www.gwu.edu/~iscopes/precproc.htm
The Integrated Health Promotion Research Kit	http://www.health.vic.gov.au/healthpromotion/downloads/integrated_health_promo.pdf
Health Promotion Planning: A Puzzle Solver for Health Promotion Forms	http://www.healthpromotion.act.gov.au/howto/needsassess/files/HP_Puzzle_Solver_BookletXX.pdf
Canadian Mental Health Promotion Toolkit	http://www.cmha.ca/mh_toolkit/intro/intro_1.htm
Interactive Domain Model Approach (IDM) to Best Practices in Health Promotion	http://www.idmbestpractices.ca/idm.ph /intro_to_IDM_22–04–02_dist.pdf
Health Promotion Project Standards	http://www.tdh.state.tx.us/php/pubs/qualhp/ProjStandard.pdf
The Programme Plan Index (PPI): An Evaluation Tool for Assessing the Quality of Adolescent Pregnancy Prevention Programme Plans	http://hpp.sagepub.com/cgi/reprint/4/4/375
Getting to Outcomes (GTO), Vol. I	http://www.stanford.edu/~davidf/GTO_Volume_I.pdf
Centre for Substance Abuse Prevention (CSAP): Building a Successful Prevention Programme	http://casat.unr.edu/bestpractices/index.htm

The website addresses for each of these tools are listed, which will not only provide you with more in-depth information on each tool, but also enable you to access and make use of them. If you can, take some time now to visit each of the tools' websites and briefly survey them, or look at the extracts from four of the best known and used tools: PRECEDE-PROCEED, Preffi, GTO and IDM.

While most of the tools address all of the planning stages with which you are familiar, many place greater emphasis on some stages than others. You will find as you familiarize yourself with these tools, that they each take a unique approach to programme planning while still incorporating the same basic stages for planning a health promotion intervention. Some are better suited for community-based interventions, while others are adapted for larger-scale programmes. The methods the tools employ to facilitate planning often differ from one another. You will find that you are more comfortable with some methods than with others. In many instances, a tool was developed for a particular type of intervention but its overall instruction is a useful aid in planning various types of programmes. The tools vary in their characteristics. Some of the main features to consider are discussed below.

Scale of intervention

The Programme Management Guidelines for Health Promotion, The Public Health Bush Book, PRECEDE-PROCEED, the Puzzle Solver and the Canadian Mental Health Promotion Toolkit are all planning tools most suitable for planning community-based programmes. This can be seen in their shared focus on cultural and environmental context and the consideration of volunteers and community engagement in the planning process. Some of the other tools listed also engage in discussions of the cultural context of interventions but maintain only a small or no focus on use of volunteers or community members in programme planning. These tools – The Integrated Health Promotion Research Kit, IDM, Health Promotion Project Standards, GTO and CSAP – place more emphasis on resource matters, collaboration between agencies and organizations, and require a more rigid structure be followed in planning. These tools are appropriate for both community-based and larger-scale programming.

Facilitation of planning

Tools vary in the way they facilitate the planning progress. While all tools provide detailed explanations of the steps they feel are most crucial in the planning process, the methods they use to facilitate that process vary from tool to tool. Some are more structured and rigid, while others are more flexible.

Use of checklists

The most common method used is explanation, coupled with checklists. Checklists are a way to ensure that you have completed all the stages that are indicated in the explanations. They allow for you to use the explanations to plan your programme and then double check that you have included the most important elements from the explanations in your planning process. Tools that utilize checklists are the Programme Management Guidelines for Health Promotion, The Public Health Bush Book, The Integrated Health Promotion Research Kit, Health Promotion Project Standards and GTO.

Assessment tools

A few of the tools are assessment tools. In some cases, they provide a brief explanation of the planning process, but the bulk of the tool is devoted to some sort of process assessment. Like the checklists, the assessment tools allow you to compare your programme plan with the points they consider most important. Assessment tools are Preffi and PPI. Preffi is a tool favoured by many health promotion professionals for its extensive assessment system, but you may find it complicated to use if you are just entering the field.

Use of forms and worksheets

A final method of facilitation of the planning process is a more open-ended method, including the use of worksheets, forms or tables. Tools using these are The Public Health Bush Book (worksheets), A Puzzle Solver (forms), IDM (forms and tables) and CSAP (worksheets). These are especially useful if you need extra guidance, since they walk you through the planning process, prompting you to complete each step by filling in a form, worksheet or table.

In Table 13.2 you will find a summary of each tool's strengths. This table also highlights some of the key differences between them. For instance, note that tools like The Public Health Bush Book and GTO have a strong emphasis on operating programmes within a cultural context. You may conclude from this information that these planning tools would be some of the most suitable to employ in planning an intervention for a target group outside of the mainstream.

Table 13.2 Summary of the strengths of selected planning tools

Planning tool	Strengths
Programme Management Guidelines for Health Promotion	Clear explanations with support from case studies and checklists Focus on sustainability
The Public Health Bush Book	Inclusion of checklists and planning and evaluation worksheets Good community development tool Attention to cultural context
Preffi 2.0	Detailed explanations with support from evidence Very strong assessment methods allowing for programme reflection and revision Includes useful planning recommendations, many important for large-scale programmes Allows for flexibility Useful in a variety of settings
PRECEDE-PROCEED	'Backwards' approach leads to thorough problem analysis Detailed evaluation process Good for community-based intervention due to emphasis on individual engagement

Table 13.2 continued

The Integrated Health Promotion Resource Kit	Use of checklists and toolkits Focus on collaboration between agencies and organizations Attends to context culturally and politically Includes advice on dissemination
Health Promotion Planning: A Puzzle Solver for Health Promotion Forms	Forms ensure documentation, allow for similar programmes to be established Complete planning process Thorough evaluation
Canadian Mental Health Promotion Toolkit	Uses case studies to explain guidance Works from the bottom up with community members Emphasis on programme planning within a specific context Effective methods for programme development Particular attention to sustainability and dissemination
IDM	Structured tables for programme planning allow for individual specificity Encourages reflection to facilitate process of ongoing programme revision Emphasis on ethics renders it suitable for more sensitive areas of health promotion
Health Promotion Project Standards	Checklists good for standardizing programmes Offers a practical planning approach Emphasis on operating a programme within contextual boundaries
PPI	Good assessment tool for project planning Emphasizes planning in context of current environment
GTO	Action steps and checklists facilitate planning Incorporates 'cultural competence' throughout Requires attention to environmental context, including examination of relevant research and evidence Strong focus on implementation, continuous improvement and sustainability
CSAP	Thorough plan formulation and evaluation guided by explanations and worksheets Provides a multitude of links to supporting resources

✏ **Activity 13.3**

Take a few minutes to find other similarities between tools. Can you draw any conclusions between what these particular strengths might mean in terms of programme planning and their application?

Feedback

Other examples of similarities that you may have noticed is the attention to needs assessment (the first stage of the planning process). The *Integrated Health Promotion Resource Kit, Canadian Mental Health Promotion Kit, Health Promotion Project Standards, PPI and GTO* all contain a strong message of operating within an appropriate environmental or political context. From this, you can see that these tools have a strong focus on programme development and would be especially useful for less experienced programme planners who have not yet become accustomed to the many factors that it is necessary to address in a needs assessment.

Another similarity you may have noticed is that some tools like the *Programme Management Guidelines* and the *Canadian Mental Health Promotion Toolkit* incorporate discussions of sustainability. Therefore, these tools may be more useful than others for planning longer-term interventions. The inclusion of community development discussions in tools like *The Public Health Bush Book, PRECEDE-PROCEED* and the *Canadian Mental Health Promotion Toolkit* show that these tools may be the most useful for planning interventions aiming to involve community members as volunteers or key actors.

In Activity 13.2, you planned your own smoking intervention based on the key stages of programme planning. To understand better the methodology of planning a health promotion intervention with the use of a planning tool, you now have the opportunity to practise with two of the planning tools discussed above: Interactive Domain Model Approach (IDM) and Getting to Outcomes (GTO).

The following is a short description of the IDM.

The IDM in brief

At its heart the IDM is very simple. When asked in workshops what influences decision making, people identify a wide sweep of factors that inevitably fall into the broad categories of values, theories, evidence and the environment (ranging from the physical to the political). These categories, including practice itself, correspond to the IDM domains and subdomains:

- The domain of *underpinnings* includes the subdomains of values/goals/ethics, theories/beliefs, and evidence; our underpinnings are our foundation, which influence us even when we are not consciously aware of how we define or prioritize them.
- The domain of *understanding of the environment* includes the subdomains of vision, analysis of health-related issues, and analysis of work-organization-related issues; our environments range from the organizations we work in to the international arena and include a variety of socio-economic and political systems and structures, and psychological and physical conditions.
- The domain of *practice* includes the subdomains of responding to health-related issues, responding to work-organization-related issues, and research (including evaluation); practice is composed of processes, activities and strategies.

As can be seen in Figure 13.1, the domains and subdomains exist in the context of the broader environment. The domains and subdomains are interactive – that is, each influences and is influenced by the others.

The IDM framework in brief

The challenge facing practitioners is, first, to identify and define our health promotion underpinnings and understanding of the environment and, second, to apply these to our practice. This is where the IDM framework comes in.

The IDM framework, the practical application of the IDM, is a multi-purpose 'change' tool for practitioners and organizations in any situation who want to pursue a best practices approach to health promotion. Using a health promotion filter to ensure that practice is consistent with health promotion underpinnings and understanding of the environment, the IDM framework can help to:

- increase understanding of health promotion, and build capacities and supports
- makes decisions and policies
- increase communication and 'team build'
- plan, implement, evaluate, and revise programmes/activities that are sensitive to local conditions
- 'make the case' for programmes/activities
- achieve health promotion goals

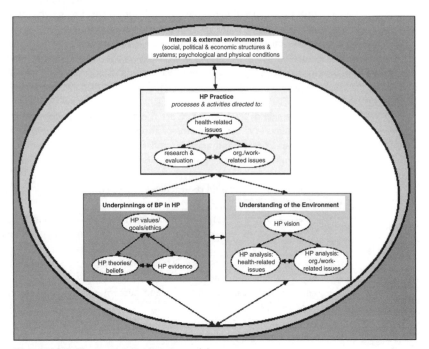

Figure 13.1 The interactive domain model

BP = best practices, HP = health promotion

Source: Kahan and Goodstadt (2002)

The framework leads us through a process where, from a health promotion perspective (that is, keeping in mind health promotion values and all the other subdomains), we answer the following questions about our activities and programmes:

- where are we now and where do we want to go?
- how do we get to where we want to go?
- what did we do, how did we do it, and what were the results?
- what do we need to change to move forward?
- what criteria and guiding principles will help us in our journey?

It does this through a series of steps, which are meant to be used 'organically' rather than linearly – that is, according to the demands of our particular situation and how we work best rather than in a set order.

As can be seen in Table 13.3, along the top of the framework are a series of steps related to preparing a foundation for action, planning and evaluation, documenting implementation (including identification of outcomes and impacts), and revision:

1 In the first set of steps we put in place a solid foundation for practice by: (a) identifying general health promotion criteria and guiding principles, (b) examining the current situation, and (c) developing a picture of our ideal situation.
2 In the second set of steps we develop an action and evaluation plan to make our picture of the ideal a reality, defining the what and how (i.e. relevant activities, tasks and processes), the who and the when, all with respect to specific objectives to achieve the ideal resources, challenges and ongoing evaluation.
3 In the third set we document what happens when the action and evaluation plan is implemented with respect to activities, processes and outcomes/impacts.
4 In the last set, based on our evaluation and documentation processes, we revise our ideal picture and/or our action and evaluation plan.

Down the side of the framework are the domains and subdomains from the IDM – that is, underpinnings (values/goals/ethics, theories/beliefs, evidence), understanding of the environment (vision and analysis) and practice (responding to issues, and research and evaluation). These act as a health promotion filter for the framework's steps.

The application of the IDM to practice involves constant questioning and reflection:

- what are our health promotion underpinnings and understanding of the environment?
- how well does our practice match our underpinnings and understanding of the environment?
- how can we increase the consistency between practice, underpinnings and understanding of the environment?
- how do our processes, activities and outcomes relate to each other, and how can we improve them?
- what resources, capacities and supports do we have to draw on, and how can we maintain and enhance them?

Table 13.3 The IDM framework

	Step 1: Prepare Foundation for Action re: selected issue			Step 2: Make Action & Evaluation Plan • how do we get to where we want to go: who does what, when & how?				Step 3: Document Implementation of Plan		Step 4: Revise
	health promotion criteria & guiding principles	current situation • where are we now?	picture of ideal situation • where do we want to go?	specific objectives to achieve ideal	resources	challenges	evaluation plan	activities & processes • what did we do? how did we do it?	outcomes of activities & processes • what were the results?	revisions • what do we need to change?
UNDERPINNINGS values goals ethics theories beliefs evidence										
UNDERSTANDING OF ENVIRONMENT vision (org/work) vision (health) analysis (org/work) analysis (health)										
PRACTICE processes/activities org/work response health response research/evaluation										

Source: Kahan and Goodstadt (2002)

Now read the following short description of the GTO.

 Features of the GTO accountability system

1 **The GTO system emphasizes accountability**
   In GTO, programme accountability involves putting a comprehensive system in place to help your programmes achieve results. That system involves asking and answering the ten accountability questions.

2 **You can use the GTO system at any stage of your work**
   We know that many practitioners are in the middle of programming and cannot begin with the first accountability question. No matter where you are in your process, the components of the Getting to Outcomes process are useful. For example, if an evidence-based programme has been chosen, planned and is being implemented, accountability questions on process and outcome evaluation and continuous quality improvement can still be valuable.

3 **GTO uses the risk and protective factor model**
   The risk and protective factor model is helpful in understanding the underlying risk conditions that contribute to the problem and the protective factors that reduce these negative effects. It has been found in many studies that these factors have been related to substance use among youth such that the more risk factors present for an individual the more likely they will be to use substances, and the more protective factors present the less likely they will be to use substances. The risk and protective factor model is organized across the domains of individual/peer, family, school and community. The factors are useful in setting up a logic model that can be used in programme planning, implementation and evaluation. In fact, these factors have been turned into variables that can be measured with surveys that are commonly available.

4 **GTO encourages the use of logic models to ensure a conceptual link between the identified problem and the potential solutions**
   It is useful to determine the most likely causes or underlying risk factors contributing to the problem and the protective factors that can be strengthened. The logic model process begins with identifying the causes or underlying factors within your community.

Overview of a logic model
A *logic* model can be defined as a series of connections that link problems and/or needs you are addressing with the actions you will take to obtain your outcomes. The programme activities should target those factors that you have identified as contributing to the problem. Logic models are frequently phrased in terms of 'if–then' statements that address the logical result of an action. For example:

- *if* prevention programmes are targeted at multiple domains (e.g. school, community and family), *then* they are more likely to produce results
- *if* alcohol, tobacco and drugs are difficult for youth to obtain, *then* youth are less likely to use them

Logic models convey very clear messages about the logic (i.e. theory) about why a programme is proposed to work. Sharing logic models early in the process with programme

Logic models convey very clear messages about the logic (i.e. theory) about why a programme is proposed to work. Sharing logic models early in the process with programme staff as well as community members is often a worthwhile activity. We have found that it helps to have a logic model diagram of how and why a programme should work.

The GTO logic model specifies four key programme elements

Needs → Goals/Objectives (risk factor-based) → Activities → Outcome Measures

Table 13.4 is an example of a logic model grid that shows how there is a direct relationship between the reasons for the problem (causes identified in a needs assessment), the desired goals and objectives to correct the problem (based on risk and protective factors), the solution to bring about those changes (i.e. the activities of a programme), and the tool (outcome measure) used to document the changes. The example is based on a real programme in a real community.

 Activity 13.4

Work through the directives of each tool separately to re-plan your intervention. You've done most of the work already. Now all you need to do is use your existing intervention and fit it into the directives of both of the tools, making adjustments to your original plan when necessary. Re-write your plan separately for each of the tools. Make sure you are using the resources given by both.

Also, think about the strengths and limitations of the tools. While IDM uses tables to guide the planning process, GTO uses checklists. Note the pros and cons of these two approaches. Was one more helpful than another in facilitating your planning process?

 Feedback

As you adjusted your plan to fit with the IDM approach, you probably had to be more specific about ethics and values throughout the planning process. Your plan should be written as a completion of the IDM tables, which highlight these underpinnings at every step. When you re-worked your plan with GTO, you should have had more of a free-standing plan written out, since GTO does not provide any items like forms or tables to complete as you go through the planning process. When using GTO, you will have found yourself thinking more about implementation, continuous improvement and sustainability, which should be reflected in your plan write-up.

In any planning process it is important to carefully document each step. In this respect, tables, like the ones used by the IDM approach, allow for thorough documentation with attention to several areas. At the same time, however, you may find these tables overwhelming because of the rigid requirements for completion. Don't forget that if you find the tables too detailed for your purposes, you can use them as a guide or adapt them more specifically to your needs. Just because a box exists in a table does not mean it must be completed.

Table 13.4 Example logic model grid

Needs assessment data	Risk-factor-based goals/objectives	Programme and activities	Outcome measures
High rate of child abuse and neglect cases in Springfield* families	Goal: Youth in Springfield's North and South neighbourhoods will have an increased rate of adult supervision during after-school hours and their parents will know their whereabouts Objective: Within the first year, 95% of PYP youth will report that their parents know their whereabouts	Positive Youth Program (PYP), Decision-Making Program (DMP), Heritage Projects • Weekly after-school youth groups, community service projects	Youth reports
Rate of confirmed child abuse and neglect cases for Springfield between 1995–96 was three times the state average	Goal: Increase parental–child attachment and social bonding Objective: Within the first year, 75% of programme youth's parents/guardians will attend biannual family celebrations. 20% improvement in measures of bonding	DMP, parent sessions • Writer and spring celebrations for youth and families	– Parent interview – Risk and protective factor survey
Springfield had a 28.3% increase in arrests for family violence from 1995–1996, which was the second highest increase in the state	Goal: Increase parental involvement Objective: Within the first year, 50% of programme youth's parents/guardians will complete the family support sessions. 20% of youth report spending more time with parents	DMP, parent sessions • Weekly telephone contact with parent or guardian by group leader	– Parent interview – Risk and protective factor survey

Source: Chinman et al. (2004)
* Names in this example have been changed

One of the main limitations of working with tables is use in a collaborative framework. It is quite time-consuming for groups of people to work on a table simultaneously. If you are planning on working in collaboration with others, it is advisable that you choose a tool that doesn't utilize tables as part of its planning process.

Checklists like those used in GTO are often preferred by many individuals because they don't appear to be as limiting as tables. In some cases, the checklists allow for more flexibility in programme planning; you can plan each stage and then confirm you have done so thoroughly by comparing your work with checklist suggestions. You may find that the checklists serve as a guide while tables are too constraining. On the other hand, you may prefer to work within the confines of a table for guidance if you feel the checklists are micro-managing your planning process.

 Activity 13.5

Now think about the usefulness of each of the tools, IDM and GTO, with regard to the type of intervention you planned. Does one tool cater to your intervention better than the other? Write down what kinds of interventions you think would be most appropriate to plan with each of the two tools.

 Feedback

The Interactive Domain Model, as noted earlier, places a heavy emphasis on ethics and values. This makes this tool more suitable for planning interventions of a sensitive nature. In some cases, this could mean planning for marginalized groups. Another way this emphasis on underpinnings can be used is in planning a large-scale programme. It is easy to lose track of these values when working out logistics such as funding and resources for an intervention operating for a large audience. Thus, using the IDM approach in planning ensures these values are not overlooked.

As mentioned in a previous section, GTO is suited to community-based, small-level programmes as well as larger-scale ones. This tool goes a long way to promote consideration of context both culturally (making this tool appropriate as a guide for planning programmes for groups who are not part of the mainstream) and also environmentally (ensuring that you will not duplicate an existing programme and have an idea of what resources and policies will have an effect on the programme).

Summary

In this chapter, you have learnt how to plan a health promotion programme or intervention. You were introduced to the basic steps in the planning process and to several tools available to assist with planning. It is hoped that you will have developed a basic understanding of the tools presented and are able to determine tools most appropriate for your particular purposes. Different tools have different strengths and limitations. Your familiarization with each tool should allow you to make an educated decision about which tool best fits your planning style or your proposed intervention.

References

Chinman M, Imm P, Wandersman A (2004) *Getting To Outcomes 2004: Promoting Accountability Through Methods and Tools for Planning, Implementation, and Evaluation*. Santa Monica, CA: Rand Health (available at: http://www.rand.org/pubs/technical_reports/2004/RAND_TR101.pdf)

Kahan B, Goodstadt M (2002) *The IDM Manual: Introduction & Basics*. Toronto: Centre for Health Promotion, University of Toronto

Evaluation of health promotion

14

Overview

The development of an evidence base relies on the availability of high-quality evaluations that can support decision makers with information about the types of programmes that should be developed and implemented to ensure the most effective use of resources. In this chapter, you will explore why evaluation is necessary, consider the current debates in the literature about the most appropriate means of evaluating health promotion and rehearse the steps required to carry out a good quality health promotion evaluation.

Learning objectives

After working though this chapter, you will be better able to:

• appreciate the importance of evaluation
• understand the political consequences of evaluation
• assess the particular problems of evaluating health promotion interventions
• distinguish between different health promotion evaluation strategies with respect to appropriateness, cost and rigour

Key terms

Attribution Being able to relate a particular outcome to a particular cause.

Effectiveness The extent to which an intervention produces a beneficial result under usual conditions.

Evaluation The process of judging the worth or value of something.

Final outcome evaluation Evaluation concerned with assessing the final outcome of a particular intervention in terms of its effect on the health of the target population.

Intermediate outcome evaluation Evaluation that focuses on the behavioural impact (intermediate outcome) of an intervention.

Process evaluation Evaluation that concentrates on examining the process of an intervention.

What is evaluation and why is it important?

There is no standard definition of evaluation. Generally, the term can be interpreted as a planned set of activities to help people see the value of their project, programme or policy. As Suchman (1967) put it, 'the process by which we judge the worth or value of something'. Evaluation tells us what is the right thing to do.

In general, evaluations should aim to:

- ensure that activities are having the intended effects (effectiveness)
- determine whether activities are cost-effective (efficiency)
- establish whether activities are acceptable to the target population (humanity)

Criteria to assess the quality of evaluations will be discussed in more detail later. However, two are crucial to the success of a good evaluation. They are the:

- *Purpose of the work*: a clear set of aims and objectives should be defined during the planning stage of the evaluation.
- *Stakeholders' perspectives*: stakeholder analysis should be carried out to understand what questions are being asked and for what purpose.

Wimbush and Watson (2000) have proposed a framework for evaluation which allows you to make explicit the specific needs (and questions being asked) and perspectives of a full range of stakeholders involved in health promotion development, implementation and practice. In doing so, they frame the types of question being asked of evaluations and the methods appropriate to producing credible evidence about the best approaches to health promotion.

 Activity 14.1

As you read the edited extracts from Wimbush and Watson's article that follows, make notes in answer to the following questions:

1 Who are the main stakeholders for health promotion evaluation?
2 What are the key stages of programme development and what is the focus of the evaluation for each stage?

 What sorts of evaluations are needed and valued?

The overall aim of evaluation is to assist people and organizations to improve their plans, policies and practices on behalf of citizens. While it is relatively easy to build consensus around evaluation for learning and improvement, there are important differences, in perspective and in emphasis, among stakeholder groups around what forms of evaluation are needed and valued. This can be illustrated with reference to the field of health promotion.

Policy makers and strategic planners

Policy makers and strategic planners need to be able to judge the effectiveness, or likely effectiveness, of health promotion programmes in order to make decisions about the most efficient and effective deployment of public resources, decisions for which they are accountable to elected representatives and citizens.

The sorts of questions they need answered are 'what works?' or 'what are the best buys?' Systematic reviews of effectiveness are intended to provide answers to such questions but tend to draw only on evidence from experimental and quasi-experimental research designs. They also require economic evaluations of health promotion interventions which look at the relationship between inputs/investments and short-term health gains.

Programme managers

Programme managers who are budget holders responsible for the delivery of health promotion programmes and local health strategies in 'real-life' circumstances need evaluations which provide feedback on the success of a range of different projects and initiatives and the extent to which they contribute to the achievement of local strategies. Here success is most likely to be assessed in terms of achieving defined objectives, reaching the targeted populations and the extent to which the local partnerships are sustainable.

Practitioners

Practitioners who are responsible for the operation and running of community health projects and services, often involving local partnership funding, find evaluations most useful when they engage with the practicalities of the implementation process, and provide feedback from people and other agencies involved in collaborative action. Evaluations which play a developmental or formative role, identifying areas for change or improvement, are particularly valued. However, those working in local projects often perceive funders' requirements for monitoring and evaluation as a 'top down' demand and struggle to cope with the multiple, duplicative and sometimes contradictory evaluation requirements of different funding bodies.

Community groups/users

The population likely to benefit from the service or programme (e.g. clients, users, the community) will be concerned with the quality of service provision, the extent to which it is relevant to their perceived needs, and the extent to which its operation is participatory or consultative. They are most likely to value evaluations which provide an avenue for feedback and involvement, address quality issues and assess community/user concerns and satisfaction. Whether an initiative delivers tangible benefits for the community is a form of effectiveness evaluation that is likely to be valued by local people, whether or not they form part of the target population.

Professional evaluators

Professional evaluators (including academic researchers) tend to engage with evaluation as a knowledge-building exercise, seeking to improve knowledge and understanding of the relationship between an intervention and its effects. They are also concerned to maintain quality standards for research, in particular with regard to research design, methodological rigour, reliability and validity.

However, evaluators employed within health promotion practice settings are often frustrated by being expected to 'evaluate everything' on a small budget and not having the resources to conduct what they regard as 'quality' research. Academic researchers are often highly critical of the quality of evaluation research carried out in practice settings, but are sometimes all too ready themselves to conduct resource-intensive evaluations of effectiveness with little attention to assuring the quality of the intervention being tested. This situation contributes to findings from large-scale evaluations which demonstrate the failure of community health interventions (e.g. Stanford, Pawtucket, Minnesota, Heartbeat Wales), the failure being attributed to the quality of programme implementation and delivery.

Inevitably, there is likely to be some overlap between the interests of the different stakeholder groups. In advocating the need for evaluation evidence that is relevant to their own particular priorities, the different stakeholder groups can disregard the necessity and contributions of other forms of evaluation. This suggests a need for more 'joined-up' thinking and partnership working on evaluation across the different stakeholder groups – policy makers and strategic planners, programme managers and practitioners, user/consumer groups – as well as those commissioning and doing evaluation work . . .

HEBS evaluation framework for health promotion

The evaluation framework developed by HEBS (1999) uses the key stages of programme development as the basis for differentiating between the types of evaluation used and useful in health promotion practice. The HEBS framework identifies the different purposes of evaluation and the associated evaluation questions that are characteristic of each of these stages, acknowledging the importance of assessing effectiveness, as well as assuring quality and making explicit the mechanisms of change implicit in a programme's theory . . .

Planning stage: systematic reviews of effectiveness

In the planning stage, once a health-related problem and the population group at risk have been identified, a second phase in the needs assessment process involves an option appraisal process which takes into account: (a) learning from other evaluation research about the most effective ways of addressing the problem with a particular group and/or within a particular setting (systematic reviews of effectiveness); (b) how the health-related need/problem is currently addressed by current policies and service provision (review of current provision/policy); (c) what professional 'experts' regard as the best ways of addressing these needs/problems (consultation interviews or seminar) . . .

Design and pilot stage: developmental evaluation

The effectiveness of interventions is increased if an initial pilot stage is undertaken before the proposed programme is fully implemented. A programme plan can be designed which is based on the initial assessment of need and appraisal of what is likely to be the most effective or 'best' intervention, given the evidence and resources available, and what can be achieved within a particular setting and set of partner agencies. Against this backdrop, the design stage involves defining the long-term goal of the programme, setting programme objectives, defining the range of activities required to meet these objectives, identifying staffing and training requirements, setting up administration, publicity and monitoring procedures.

Developmental evaluation is an essential part of this design stage. Formative evaluation is likely to be the most appropriate approach since the prime purpose of the evaluation is developmental and the process is iterative, providing continuing feedback from key stakeholders and the target group/project users in order to adjust, refine and optimize the programme's focus, design and ultimate effectiveness. If the programme is found at this stage to be unfeasible or impracticable without major revisions, then the project should be abandoned and a new approach devised . . .

Implementation stage (early start-up): monitoring and review

For evaluation purposes, it is helpful to distinguish between different phases of implementation: early start-up, establishment and a fully operational phase. Overall, the implementation stage is characterized by the operation of the full programme across all sites in its revised post-pilot form. The main tasks here are project management, quality assurance and evaluation.

At the start of a project, the project manager is concerned with defining appropriate milestones for the project, reviewing cycles and agreeing with key stakeholders appropriate performance indicators and quality standards for the project. Monitoring and review systems should be set up to continue throughout the duration of the project's life for both evaluation and quality assurance purposes. These systems include:

- monitoring systems for routinely recording data about inputs, outputs, project activities and any agreed quality standards;

- evaluation work should begin by looking at management issues around the delivery of the project and quality assurance. If the impacts and outcomes of the project are to be assessed over time, it may be appropriate to collect baseline information at this early stage.

Implementation stage (establishment): impact evaluation

This phase of implementation is when the project has become stable, project staff have gained experience and confidence and early problems have been addressed.

At this stage, 'impact evaluation' is appropriate and the evaluation focus turns to examining the implementation process: the extent to which the project is working as planned; how far the project has reached the target population; and the immediate effects of the project (i.e. its impacts or results) on the target population and others. If monitoring data on costs is available, simple economic evaluation measures such as cost effectiveness and/or cost:benefit ratio might also be produced.

Implementation stage (fully operational): outcome evaluation

Once the project is well established, the evaluation can focus on effectiveness – whether the end results, or intermediate outcomes, are being achieved and thus the extent to which the project has been effective in contributing to longer-term health and social policy goals. Outcome evaluation should be conducted when an impact evaluation has already demonstrated a programme's short-term effectiveness, ideally in several settings/populations, but long-term effectiveness is still unknown. To allow long-term follow-up over time, this type of evaluation requires dedicated and substantial research resources and those with specialist evaluation expertise who can advise on appropriate research designs and methods, implement these and conduct the appropriate analysis. One of the biggest problems with this form of evaluation is providing evidence of a causal link between the project being evaluated and the outcome measures. Experimental and quasi-experimental research designs go some way towards addressing this problem, although these designs are regarded by many as a research design that is neither feasible nor desirable for community-based interventions . . .

Dissemination stage: transfer evaluation

The dissemination stage begins when there is information available for dissemination beyond the immediate audience of project staff, funders and stakeholders, about the 'results' of, or learning from, the impact and outcome evaluation research. Typically, this is when the initial project funding period comes to an end.

Programmes that have proven to be effective will only have significant impact if they are disseminated and taken up more widely. This is the purpose of 'demonstration projects'. The focus of evaluation at this stage is on the transferability of the programme and the replicability and sustainability of its outcomes when transferred to a wider range of settings and/or populations.

 Feedback

1 You should have identified that there are a range of stakeholders who are interested in the results of evaluation, distinguishing between: policy makers; strategic planners; programme managers; practitioners; community groups/users and professional evaluators.

2 Wimbush and Watson put forward a framework for helping to isolate the evaluation methods required for each stage of the health promotion programme. These are planning, design and pilot, implementation, dissemination. You should have identified the types of questions being asked at each stage of the evaluation.

Current debates and issues in health promotion evaluation

Much has been written over the last 10 years about the most appropriate means of evaluating the work of health promotion. During the 1980s, increasing expectation within public services towards evidence-based decision making led to a desire from those working in the field of health promotion to establish a credible scientific basis for their work. Early attempts to summarize the evidence of 'what works' borrowed methodologies employed by biomedicine to systematically review evaluations of the effectiveness of health promotion interventions. The results of some recent reviews will be presented and discussed in Chapter 15.

Traditionally, a systematic review process was used to assess evaluations in terms of their methodological merit and, where appropriate, techniques such as statistical meta-analysis used, in order to pool the results of several studies focusing on a common topic, thereby gaining a more comprehensive understanding of the relevant issues. This rigorous approach is controversial, particularly on the issue of what constitutes an acceptable standard of evaluation, and thus what can be said to be 'proven' to be effective. There may be many effective interventions in place already which cannot prove their effectiveness in a systematic review due to the criteria used for assessing the quality of their evaluation. Often there is no evaluation at all and even where there is the methodological quality may be poor.

The findings from reviews of scientific studies highlight the tensions inherent in searching for the limited amount of health promotion that has been evaluated or will fit into the biomedical model of evidence. Some of the key questions include:

• What counts as evidence?
• How do certain perspectives on evidence limit the focus of our endeavours in evaluating the impact of health promotion?

- What kinds of explanatory models might help us to ask better questions?
- What does this mean for indicators of outcome in evaluation studies?

These questions have been considered by a WHO Working Group (1998), who have put forward a set of core features for the evaluation of health promotion. They are:

1 *Participation*. Each stage of evaluation should involve, in appropriate ways, those who have a legitimate interest in the initiative. Those with an interest can include: policy makers, community members and organizations, health and other professionals, and local and national health agencies. It is especially important that members of the community whose health is being addressed be involved in evaluation.
2 *Multiple methods*. Evaluation should draw on a variety of disciplines and methods.
3 *Capacity building*. Evaluations should enhance the capacity of individuals, communities, organizations and governments to address important health promotion concerns.
4 *Appropriateness*. Evaluations should be designed to accommodate the complex nature of health promotion interventions and their long-term impact. Evaluations premised on these principles provide an appropriate means of assessing and understanding health promotion initiatives.

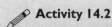 **Activity 14.2**

As you read the following extracts from the WHO Working Group report, make notes on the main differences between health promotion interventions and biomedical interventions. You will need to consider: the time frame; the end points; the nature of the intervention; who instigates the intervention; the health of the target audience; the likely size of any benefit; and the aim of the intervention.

 Evaluation of health promotion initiatives

Conclusion 1. Those who have a direct interest in a health promotion initiative should have the opportunity to participate in all stages of its planning and evaluation.

... Participation by those with a direct interest in a health promotion initiative is an important prerequisite for the evaluation of health promotion programmes and policies. Such participation increases the relevance and credibility of evaluation results, as well as the likelihood that the results will be used. In addition, participatory approaches to evaluation help foster the process of empowerment and build stake-holders' capacity to address health needs, thus giving them more control over the factors affecting their health.

Ideally, participation should extend beyond those who are the primary focus of health promotion initiatives, to include others who have a direct stake in the initiatives. These additional stakeholders include: health promotion practitioners, community representatives, policymakers, and evaluators.

Substantial evidence indicates that the results of programme evaluations are more likely to be implemented when key stakeholders have participated in all stages of the evaluation process.

The participation of stakeholder groups makes the values underlying the evaluation explicit, and allows the issues of different groups to be addressed. This, in turn, helps to increase the credibility and subsequent use of evaluation results.

The evaluation of health promotion initiatives benefits from pooling professional and lay resources, including the unique knowledge possessed by non-professionals. In addition, a participatory approach to the evaluation of health promotion grounds evaluation indicators in practical reality, and ensures that information gained through evaluation benefits all participants.

Most importantly, participatory evaluation encourages collaboration between different sectors, forcing conscious choices and a multisectoral approach to selecting indicators in complex health promotion projects. Finally, participatory evaluation provides a practical way to cross boundaries between theory and practice.

Conclusion 2. Adequate resources should be devoted to the evaluation of health promotion initiatives.

To maximize the benefits of an evaluation, budgets for health promotion initiatives must include sufficient funding for a thorough examination of their main features. The importance of adequate funding has been recognized by a number of jurisdictions, where minimum standards for the allocation of financial resources to the evaluation of health promotion programmes have been established. These have ranged from 8% to 15% of the total programme budget Analysis of previous experience supports the Working Group's view that the allocation of 10% of total programme resources is a reasonable standard to ensure the development and implementation of appropriate evaluations in health promotion. This does not, however, preclude the allocation of additional resources when necessary.

Conclusion 3. Health promotion initiatives should be evaluated in terms of their processes as well as their outcomes.

The evaluation of health promotion initiatives requires evaluation methods to assess both the process and contextual aspects of the activities, in addition to evaluation of outcomes.

Outcome-focused evaluations predominate in the current public health system. In many instances, outcome measures provide an important contribution to understanding the impact of health promotion initiatives. Outcome measures are not, however, a sufficient means of understanding the ways in which a health promotion programme or policy has brought about change.

Although outcome measures can reveal if a programme works (or does not work), they are neither intended nor designed to reveal why or how a programme works. Understanding why or how a health promotion initiative fosters change is as important as knowing whether a desired change took place, particularly when broader implementation of an initiative is planned or the context of an initiative changes significantly.

Process evaluation, combined with indicators of short- and long-term outcomes, provide the range of information needed fully to assess and understand the impact of health promotion initiatives, and make appropriate programme decisions.

Conclusion 4. The use of randomized control trials to evaluate health promotion initiatives is, in most cases, inappropriate, misleading and unnecessarily expensive.

A multidimensional focus on the determinants of health and the impossibility of imposing tight environmental controls, or their unacceptability, are inherent features of most health promotion initiatives. The randomized controlled trial is often an inappropriate and potentially misleading means of evaluating these efforts. For a better understanding of the impact of health promotion initiatives, evaluators need to use a wide range of qualitative and quantitative methods that extend beyond the narrow parameters of randomized controlled trials.

Randomized controlled trials are most effective when the intervention can be delivered and received in a standard way: that is, when variations in delivery and acceptance are minimized. Health promotion programmes can vary greatly in both of these dimensions. Variability may occur, first, in the delivery of an information campaign, implementation of a school programme or enforcement of a policy, and, second, in audience attention to or acceptance of campaign messages or participation in a programme. In addition, because health promotion is often a long-term process, frequently involving environmental modifications, attempts to keep environmental conditions constant can undermine the processes that health promotion attempts to influence.

Conclusion 5. Expertise in the evaluation of health promotion initiatives needs to be developed and sustained.

As with other scientific activities, the evaluation of health promotion initiatives requires specific skills and capacities. Given the diverse nature of health promotion programmes and policies, these skills extend beyond the domain of health sciences to include social science methods, organizational change theory, participatory action research and other approaches to knowledge development that are compatible with core health promotion principles and values.

At present, the field of health promotion lacks both an adequate infrastructure to develop expertise in evaluation and evaluators with the knowledge and skills to make appropriate assessments. This deficit, in many instances, has resulted in the adoption of inappropriate criteria for evaluating health promotion initiatives.

To ensure that evaluators possess the requisite skills for examining health promotion initiatives, the capacity for monitoring and evaluation must be supported and strengthened at every level of policy-making. This requires the establishment of a strategy for the development and maintenance of an adequate infrastructure for the development of skills in the evaluation of health promotion initiatives, as well as the dissemination of information about appropriate evaluation methods.

↻ Feedback

1 *Long-term versus short-term outcomes.* Health promotion is concerned with long-term as opposed to short-term outcomes. For example, if you encourage a young person to take up exercise, this may be to prevent heart disease that might occur thirty or forty years later. In health care, you might carry out a heart bypass operation and the outcome of the operation would be known in a few months and even long-term outcomes would be known within a few years.

2 *Health promotion endpoints are rare – in health care they are common.* Most of the population are not going to die of the specific disease that health promoters are focusing on. Consider the example of accident prevention: most people are not going to die in accidents.

3 *Health promotion involves public policy.* Decisions about how to implement health promotion interventions are largely the result of public policy, whereas health care involves clinical decisions made by the individual practitioners.

4 *Health promotion is imposed.* Health promotion is initiated or imposed, whereas clinical treatment is demand-led, in that the patient is sick and seeks help. People do not usually ask for health promotion.

5 *Health promotion works with healthy clients.* Related to the last point, in clinical settings people are ill and therefore are more likely to comply with an intervention and see it to be beneficial. In the case of health promotion, people are well and therefore the benefits of an intervention, especially if the outcomes cannot be seen for thirty or forty years, are unlikely to be important for that person at that point in time.

6 *Health promotion has a small proportional benefit.* Perhaps the biggest problem stems from the fact that the benefit to the individual of health promotion activities is very small, although the benefit to the population as a whole can be great. However, in the case of health care, the benefit of treating a person who is ill may be very large to that individual, but small to society.

7 *Health promotion operates in a different paradigm.* The use of similar methods of evaluation of health care and for health promotion may not be justified.

What are the different approaches to evaluation and when should we use them?

There is no single, correct way to evaluate – instead, the method that is most appropriate will depend on the aims and objectives of the intervention, the types of information or data available, and the time and resources available. However, it is important to note that there are two main research ideologies that often lead health promotion professionals to choose the wrong method for their evaluation. The two, often opposing, research methodologies put forward in the debate about the evaluation of health promotion are:

1 The positivist approach which usually advocates a quantitative approach:
   • the assumption that it is possible to generate objective accounts of the world
   • an attempt to describe general patterns and account for causal relationships and general laws
   • the idea that there is a unity of methods between the natural and the social sciences
   • the use of scientific method for testing hypotheses

2 A phenomenological tradition which underpins a qualitative approach:
   • individuals interpret and make sense of their world
   • access to knowledge happens by gaining access to these subjective understandings

Much time is wasted in debating the relative merits of these perspectives on evaluation. The golden rule, therefore, is to choose the right method for answering the questions posed by the users of the evaluation results. These may involve choosing a mix of qualitative and quantitative methods.

Evaluations may focus on one or more of three aspects of an intervention: the processes; the intermediate outcome; and the final outcome.

Process evaluation

Process evaluation is about assessing the effect of an intervention in terms of the processes. Examples of the type of question that a process evaluation deals with include:

- Is the programme reaching the target group? (That would require a quantitative study)
- Are participants satisfied with the programme? (Could be qualitative or quantitative)
- Are the activities of the programme being implemented as planned?

Process evaluation allows useful insights into the implementation process, for example how interventions are interpreted and responded to by different groups. However, in general, process evaluation is most useful when carried out in conjunction with outcome evaluation.

Intermediate outcome evaluation

This type of evaluation can be carried out immediately after an intervention, to look at the intermediate outcomes (rather than the final outcomes – see below). It is a popular method of evaluation. Outcome evaluations use either randomized or non-randomized studies such as cohort and case-control studies. Their focus tends to be on the behavioural impact of a particular intervention. The types of question that it deals with includes:

- what proportion of the target group has heard of the health promotion activities?
- Has there been a change in behaviour, for example more people exercising?

Final outcome evaluation

This, as the name suggests, is concerned with assessing the long-term effects or consequences on the health of the target audience (e.g. a lower rate of lung cancer in people exposed to anti-smoking advice). Because of the time lag between an intervention and the final outcome, this type of evaluation is complex to carry out and costly.

The design which is commonly advocated for evaluations of final outcomes is the randomized controlled trial, despite its lack of fit with the principles and the range of activities employed in health promotion. Randomized controlled trials are widely considered as the 'gold standard' in the clinical field because of their high internal validity (i.e. the most rigorous means of establishing a clear relationship between an intervention and a health outcome). However, there are some problems in using randomized controlled trials to evaluate health promotion, as explained in the following edited extracts from an article by Nutbeam (1998).

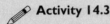

Activity 14.3

As you read the extracts, make notes in answer to the following questions:

1   What are the advantages and disadvantages of using the randomized control trial as
    a means of evaluating health promotion activities?
2   What types of methods are available for measuring the success of health promotion
    programmes and what are their limitations?
3   What can be done to improve the quality of evaluations in health promotion?

Evaluation of outcome: assessing cause and effect

It is hard to identify a simple causal chain which links a health promotion action to changes
in health status. Such a simplistic 'reductionist' model for health promotion and disease
prevention has long been discredited. The link between health promotion action and
eventual health outcomes is usually complex and difficult to trace – a fact which poses real
dilemmas in evaluations which seek to use social and health outcomes as primary measures of 'success'.

For example, smoking is a major cause of illness and disability which threatens the quality
of life of many people. Quitting smoking or never starting will greatly reduce the future
incidence and prevalence of several major causes of premature death, disease and disability.
But even here, where the link between a behaviour and health outcome is clearly established, the relationship between different forms of health promotion intervention – education, behavioural counselling, changing social attitudes, environmental restrictions and price
increases – and subsequent decisions by an individual to quit or not to start, are very
complex. Where the relationship is less well established or acknowledged – for example
the relationship between income distribution or employment status and health (Kaplan et
al., 1996) – defining a causal chain between actions designed to alleviate the health impact
of these determinants, and subsequent health outcomes becomes even more problematic.
Currently, far more attention is being given to the complexities of these relationships, and
the implications for public health action to respond to them. Given this situation, great
attention needs to be given to clarity in the definition of health promotion outcomes, and
to the evidence which indicates their relation to intermediate health outcomes, and subsequent health and social outcomes. Based on this model, evaluation of health promotion
action should be based on measurement of change in the three types of health promotion
outcome – achievement of improved personal health literacy, changes to public policies
and organisational practices, and changes to social norms and community actions which,
individually or in combination, increase people's control over the determinants of health.

In assessing the outcome to an intervention, two basic questions have to be addressed,
namely:

(i)   can change be observed in the object of interest; and
(ii) can this observed change be attributed to the intervention?

. . . the basic principles of study design are considered here, along with a small number of
issues which are of greatest relevance to the evaluation of health promotion programmes.

Attribution of cause and effect: experimental designs and their problems
. . . Unfortunately, meeting the basic criteria for the randomised design has proved difficult and often runs counter to the valued processes in health promotion concerning

participation in decision-making (Allison and Rootman, 1996). Though some studies have successfully employed this design, most have been narrowly defined, typically restricted to single issues (e.g. smoking), single health promotion objectives (e.g. improving health literacy, changing health behaviour), and interventions undertaken in highly manageable, 'closed' systems such as schools, health clinics, and workplaces . . .

These studies are important in advancing knowledge and building credibility for health promotion but, for community-based and communitywide programmes, they may be too restrictive, and may ultimately be self-defeating by reducing the effectiveness of the intervention or rendering it impossible to reproduce (Black, 1996). Alternative approaches have to be identified.

Alternatives to experimental design
In circumstances where, for practical reasons (often financial) there are no opportunities to establish a reference population, additional strategies to strengthen inference about programme effects have been developed. These include monitoring changes over time in the object of interest, referred to as a 'time series design'. This is the simplest and least obtrusive form of evaluation. It can often involve use of existing methods of record-keeping; for example, monitoring change in the use of a screening service before, during and after a programme to promote improved uptake; phasing the introduction of interventions into different communities, and observing a change in the intervention population in equivalent phases related to the introduction of the intervention. Such a design temporarily creates a 'non-intervention' population. This is a useful design to overcome the ethical dilemma of deliberately withholding an intervention to a study population. It does not so easily allow for detection of longer-term effects of interventions as a traditional experimental or quasi-experimental design. Differing intervention intensity in different populations is particularly feasible when an intervention consists of different elements (e.g. organisational change, personal education, mass media education). The programme can be offered as a whole to one population, while, by contrast, only the individual component parts are offered to other populations . . .

Strategic issues in evaluating community/population interventions
Beyond these technical solutions, there is a more fundamental and strategic problem in the use of experimental designs in the evaluation of health promotion programmes. In interventions which are designed to influence human behaviour and social interactions, the artificial assignment of individuals in communities to intervention and control groups is not only often impractical, but frequently impossible as it places quite unrealistic constraints on the intervention design. For example, it is virtually impossible to use the mass media in such a way that the intervention only reaches a randomly selected population group. Further, many health promotion programmes actively draw upon political systems and community networks as part of the intervention. In such circumstances the 'random' allocation of individuals would place impossible constraints on the possibility of actively using community networks.

As well as these practical constraints, interventions have been strategically designed to influence populations rather than individuals . . . The cardiovascular health promotion programmes provide a good example of efforts to overcome many of the practical problems for evaluation design in programmes directed at whole populations as opposed to individuals. The cardiovascular programmes sought to modify traditional experimental designs in ways which suited the practicalities of the interventions being organised. Whole populations were the 'unit' of intervention, and were matched with equivalent comparison 'units', geographically isolated from the intervention. Thus, the community was the unit of assignment, but the individual remained the unit of observation.

This quasi-experimental design has become the norm for such programmes and has been widely promoted as the best approach to evaluation of community-based programmes. An enhanced version of this quasi-experimental design, the community intervention trial, advocates identification of a large number of separate community 'units' and random allocation of these to intervention and control groups. This evaluation design has been adopted in several well-known studies in the past decade and is considered by some to be the 'only design appropriate for the evaluation of lifestyle interventions that cannot be allocated to individuals' (Murray, 1995).

Community interventions and social movements
Despite this technical progress in developing suitable evaluation designs for well-defined population interventions, the results from the cardiovascular programmes and from the COMMIT smoking cessation trial – the largest experiment with a community intervention trial design – have generally been considered disappointing in terms of their observable net impact on targeted risks. In most cases, positive results have been seen in both intervention and comparison communities. Explanations of these results not only consider the possibility that the interventions may have been insufficiently intense, too brief, or failed to penetrate a sufficient proportion of the population to have had an impact over and above prevailing 'secular trends', but also that the study designs may not have been as useful or sensitive as required for such complex interventions (Mittelmark et al., 1993; Susser, 1995; Fisher, 1995). In addition, some commentators have pointed to poor understanding of the broad research base for interventions (highlighted above), and emphasised the need for 'creative, dedicated, and rigorous social research' to bring about this understanding (Susser, 1995).

One explanation for observed positive results in both intervention and comparison populations is that there has been a high level of 'contamination' between the artificially separated populations. There is good evidence to suggest that this has occurred in some cases (Nutbeam et al., 1993) . . .

The WHO-sponsored programmes, such as the Healthy Cities Project and the Health Promoting Schools Project, are more often depicted as social movements than as tangible 'interventions' of the type described in the cardiovascular programmes (Tsouros, 1995). Social movements take longer to develop, and are less tangible and predictable (and therefore less easily measured and controlled by conventional means) than organized interventions. This is because they draw upon multiple forms of intervention (education, advocacy, facilitation of social mobilisation), often engage the population affected far more directly in decision-making, and rely to a certain extent on opportunism to guide the direction and emphasis of activities. Such an approach to health promotion appears more capable of addressing some of the underlying social and economic determinants of health which require sustained activism, and to offer greater opportunity for community control and empowerment – some of the more important and valued processes and outcomes in health promotion – but is impractical to evaluate using the tightly defined criteria of experimental design.

The dilemma emerging from this analysis is that the more powerful forms of health promotion action are those which appear to be longterm and least easily predicted, controlled and measured by conventional means. Against this, important and valued advances in knowledge and credibility have come from more tightly defined and controlled interventions, which have been evaluated through the application of experimental designs . . .

Building evidence using multiple methods and multiple sources of data
Qualitative public health research can provide depth and insight into people's experiences, and the social contexts that strengthen, support or diminish health. This knowledge and insight is important in explaining observed success or failure in any given programme, and essential for the successful replication and dissemination of new ideas.

Despite this, qualitative research is generally undervalued and under used. Part of the reason for this stems from a value system which has evolved among public health researchers (especially those with substantial training in epidemiology and biostatistics) which gives quantitative, experimental research high status, and tends to devalue the importance of research to determine the process of change which may often be qualitative – frequently referred to as 'soft' research. This may be because the methods involved in qualitative research may be less well defined and in many cases simply unfamiliar to researchers used to experimental designs. As a consequence, such methods may either be inappropriately applied or, when properly applied, inappropriately assessed through academic peer review . . .

One promising approach to the use of multiple methods is the concept of research 'triangulation' to improve confidence in research findings. This approach is now well established among qualitative researchers, and involves accumulating evidence from a variety of sources. The logic of this approach is that the more consistent the direction of the evidence produced from different sources, the more reasonable it is to assume that the programme has produced the observed effects. Triangulation simply means using more than one approach to answer the same question . . .

The use of 'triangulation' has much merit in the evaluation of health promotion, especially where experimental research design may be inappropriate, impractical, or provide only part of the picture in a multi-level intervention. Combining information from different quantitative and qualitative sources to assess for consistency in results can provide powerful evidence of success, as well as providing insight to the processes of change in populations and organisations.

 Feedback

1 Randomized controlled trials (RCTs) provide the best method of dealing with issues of attribution (i.e. the assessment of the effect on a desired health outcome by an intervention). However, there are many problems associated with using RCTs for evaluating health promotion: the principles of the design run counter to the values of health promotion and health promotion attempts to influence systems or populations which are difficult to randomize. However, limitations of the RCT design for many complex health promotion interventions should not be seen as an excuse for not evaluating. Much can be learned from the principles of RCTs, including: using a representative sample of the population; use of some form of pre and post assessment of objects of intervention; use of some form of control process; clear documentation of process to ensure transparency of methods.

2 There are a range of methods available for measuring the success of health promotion. The best available evidence will be derived from a range of different study designs

and methodologies. The effectiveness of health promotion should be assessed using a range of process and outcome information.

3 Standards and quality of health promotion evaluations can be improved if we are clear about the definitions of success (distinguishing between health outcomes and the outcomes of health promotion); who the stakeholders are (i.e. who is interested in the results); appropriate methods used for evaluating each stage of the health promotion process; use of triangulation of methods.

What does a good quality evaluation look like?

There are a number of steps in the process of evaluation. These are the starting points for tailoring an evaluation to the particular initiative under consideration. The steps are interdependent and although they might not be encountered in a strictly linear sequence, there is an order for the fulfilling of each – earlier steps provide the foundation for later ones. It is recommended that each of the six steps listed below should be taken in any evaluation:

1 *What are the aims and objectives of my project?* Re-visit your original plans and objectives for the project or programme. Think about how these could be measured, before, after and during your project – turn your aims and objectives into research questions, and your research questions into a plan of how you will measure your success or effectiveness. Also, consider what the wider impact of your project might be and how this might best be assessed – for example, a community café project might aim to improve the diet of a particular community group, but it might also have knock-on effects such as stronger friendships and relationships within the community that may be equally beneficial to health and well-being.

2 *What are my research questions?* The type of questions that you ask about the outcomes, processes and effects of your project will determine the 'indicators' (success or process measures) and also the research methods that you choose. If you are mostly concerned with 'how many', 'how often' or 'how much' types of questions, then you will probably choose to assess the answers to these questions with quantitative research methods – in other words, take counts of frequency, degree of change, or whatever numbers you want to assess. If, on the other hand, you are more interested in simply 'how', 'why' and more open-ended types of questions, you will probably find that choosing a qualitative method – semi-structured interviews, participant observation or focus groups, for example – will allow you the flexibility to explore these issues.

3 *How was this project expected to work?* A lot of the best projects and evaluations are carried out with a strong *theoretical* approach behind them – in other words, project managers and evaluators have thought through the 'model' or approach to health change and development that sits behind their project, and focused their evaluation questions accordingly. For example, the team behind the community café project mentioned above could be basing their hopes for the project's success on the assumptions that changing the opportunities and environment of their community group to eat healthy meals will improve their health, but also that providing this new setting will strengthen community

bonds and networks – a socio-ecological approach to health development (Thorogood and Coombes, 2000).

4 *What do I want my evaluation to do?* If you are mostly concerned with looking at the processes surrounding the set-up and implementation of a project or programme, then you will probably want to carry out a process or formative evaluation. If, on the other hand, you want to look at final outcomes of your project (against your original aims and objectives), you will probably carry out an outcome or summative evaluation.

5 *Who are the main groups and individuals involved in this project?* A good evaluation will reflect the settings, relationships and partnerships within which a project or programme has been based. When looking at the broad impact and scope of your project, think also about factors like promotion of local partnerships.

6 *Who is my evaluation for?* When you are designing your evaluation, a further thing to consider is the audience to whom you will present or publish your findings. Community groups and partners may be interested in qualitative, as well as quantitative, data. Project funders may sometimes (but not always) find quantitative data most persuasive. Think about ways of disseminating your findings. This is particularly important with community-based projects, where project users can be said to be 'stakeholders' in your endeavour. Wide and accessible dissemination is a chance for project and evaluation staff to give something back to the community that they have just 'researched', and may also provide them with an opportunity to get involved in future project plans.

 Activity 14.4

Use what you have learnt in this chapter to produce an ideal evaluation framework for a complex health promotion intervention. You may wish to use a health promotion programme known to you and critique its existing evaluation framework and make suggestions for its improvements.

 Feedback

An ideal evaluation framework should have considered and included the following steps: clear rationale and overview of the purpose of the evaluation; consideration of the methodologies required to evaluate the programme; clear set of aims and objectives of the programme and for the evaluation; a list of indicators required to measure progress of the programme; clarity about how the results of the information will be used and explicit plans to disseminate and act on the results of the findings.

Summary

You have learnt that there are a number of issues and dilemmas associated with the evaluation of health promotion. Theoretical issues surround the problem of how to measure health, particularly as our concept of health may change as we work with different communities and individuals. Practical issues are associated with the methodology used to obtain information and how this is then used or measured. Evaluators have problems in deciding what they need to measure but more importantly they have problems trying to attribute the health outcome to a specific health promotion intervention.

References

Allison KR, Rootman I (1996) Scientific rigour and community participation in health promotion research: are they compatible?, *Health Promotion International* 11: 333–40

Black N (1996) Why we need observational studies to evaluate the effectiveness of health care, *British Medical Journal* 312: 1215–18

Fisher EB (1995) The results of the COMMIT Trial, *American Journal of Public Health* 85: 159–60

Hawe P, Degeling D, Hall J (1990) *Evaluating Health Promotion: A Health Workers' Guide*. MacLennan and Petty.

Health Education Board for Scotland (1999) *Research for a Healthier Scotland: The Research Strategy of the Health Education Board for Scotland*. Edinburgh: HEBS.

Kaplan, GA, Pamuk ER, Lynch JW *et al.* (1996) Inequality in income and mortality in the US: analysis of mortality and potential pathways, *British Medical Journal* 312: 999–1003

Mittelmark MB, Hunt MK, Heath GW, Schmid TL (1993) Realistic outcomes: lessons from community based research and demonstration programs for the prevention of cardiovascular diseases, *Journal of Public Health Policy* 14: 455–62

Murray DM (1995) Design and analysis of community trials: lessons from the Minnesota Heart Health Program, *American Journal of Epidemiology* 142: 569–75

Nutbeam D (1998) Evaluating health promotion – progress, problems and solutions, *Health Promotion International* 13: 27–44 (available at: http://heapro.oupjournals.org/cgi/content/abstract/13/1/27)

Nutbeam D, Smith C, Murphy S, Catford J (1993) Maintaining evaluation designs in long-term community based health promotion programs, *Journal of Epidemiology and Community Health* 47: 123–7

Suchman EA (1967) *Evaluative Research*. New York: Russell Sage Foundation

Susser M (1995) The tribulations of trials: intervention in communities, *American Journal of Public Health* 85: 158

Thorogood M, Coombes Y (2000) *Evaluating Health Promotion: Practice and Methods*. Oxford: Oxford University Press

Tsouros AG (1995) The WHO Healthy Cities Project: state of the art and future plans, *Health Promotion International* 10: 133–41

Wimbush E, Watson J (2000) An evaluation framework for health promotion: theory, quality and effectiveness, *Evaluation* 6(63): 301–21

World Health Organization (1998) *Health Promotion Evaluation: Recommendations to Policy Makers*. Report of the WHO European Working Group on Health Promotion Evaluation. Copenhagen: WHO (available at: http://www.who.dk/document/e60706.pdf)

Further reading

Campbell M *et al.* (2000) Framework for design and evaluation of complex interventions to improve health, *British Medical Journal* 321: 694–6 (available at: http://bmj.bmj-journals.com/cgi/reprint/321/7262/694)

Hills D (2004) *Evaluation of Community-level Interventions for Health Improvement: A Review of Experience in the UK*. London: Health Development Agency (available at: http://www.publichealth.nice.org.uk/documents/community_review.pdf)

Naidoo J, Wills J (2000) *Health Promotion: Foundations for Practice*, 2nd edn. London: Ballière Tindall/Royal College of Nursing Publications

World Health Organization (2001) *Evaluation in Health Promotion. Principles and Perspectives.* WHO Regional Publications European Series, #92. Copenhagen: WHO

15

Evidence-based health promotion

Overview

In this final chapter, you will learn how the ideas of taking an evidence-based approach may be applied in health promotion. The principles of the approach are outlined, the problems associated with the application of evidence-based approaches are considered, and the gap between practice and evidence is noted. Two examples of an evidence base for health promotion are presented, with a description of the main findings and their implications for health promotion practice.

Learning objectives

When you have completed this chapter, you should be able to:

- **describe the need for an evidence base in health**
- **understand the practical and methodological challenges in developing an evidence base**
- **understand the challenge of getting research into practice**

Key terms

Evidence-based medicine Movement in the medicine and related professions to base clinical practice on the most rigorous scientific basis, principally informed by the results of randomized controlled trials of the effectiveness of interventions.

Evidence-based practice The use of research evidence to guide practice, often associated with, but not synonymous with, the development of guidelines.

Evidence into practice The attempt to implement evidence in practice.

Introduction

Towards the end of the twentieth century, there emerged in many high-income countries an appetite for taking an evidence-based approach to policy (Davies *et al.*, 2000). This idea took its lead from developments in evidence-based medicine, where a systematic approach to using research evidence in clinical medicine had been underway for about thirty years. *Effectiveness and Efficiency: Random Reflections on Health Services*, written by Archie Cochrane in 1972, set out a number of principles which he argued ought to be applied to clinical medicine. These were that there had to be some means of determining the cost-effectiveness of health care interventions so that ineffective and harmful practice could be eliminated. Note that when Cochrane made these proposals they were seen as very radical as far as clinical medicine was concerned. In the past decade, it has become equally important to ensure that health promotion is also evidence based.

Challenges in developing evidence-based health promotion

Six issues need to be considered when building the evidence base for health promotion. First, there is the conundrum at the heart of public health. This is that while health at an aggregate level in high-income countries has improved throughout the last century and a half, in the last forty years or so inequalities between socio-economic groups have widened, with the difference between the most and least advantaged the most pronounced (Graham and Kelly, 2004). In other words, things have been getting better and worse simultaneously.

Second, evidence of the effectiveness of interventions to reduce health inequalities is poor. Less than 0.5 per cent of published papers by British researchers in public health deal with intervention research (Millward *et al.*, 2003). There is also a real paucity of information on the cost-effectiveness of interventions, or indeed cost data, to allow calculations of cost-effectiveness to be done (Wanless, 2004).

Third, of the evidence that does exist, there is more about 'downstream' interventions rather than upstream interventions. In other words, there is an emphasis in the literature on things like individually based interventions for promoting physical activity, rather than about the environmental factors like traffic and parks which might promote physical activity (Hillsdon *et al.*, 2004).

Fourth, as discussed in Chapter 5 on the determinants of health, empirical descriptions of the social variations in populations are underdeveloped in most countries. This is important because social variations are important mediating factors in the ways that different segments of the population respond to interventions. Socio-economic categories for describing populations are still primarily organized around occupations and, important though these are for providing aggregate accounts of mortality at the population level, they lack sufficient detail and fail to take account of the importance of cultural and social factors that have an impact on health (Graham and Kelly, 2004).

 Activity 15.1

The fifth issue relates to the nature of research evidence. As you have seen in Chapter 14, the effectiveness literature is dominated by use of the randomized controlled trial. Why does this present a problem for health promotion?

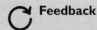 **Feedback**

This is not a problem at one level because it is the right type of study design for determining effectiveness. However, its very power creates a knock on effect with respect to the hierarchy of evidence. In other words, because the randomized controlled trial (RCT) is so good at what it does, if it is done properly, some commentators at least see evidence derived from other sources as inferior. This is not helpful, because while RCTs are good on internal validity, they tend to be much less informative about issues of process and implementation, which are vital to know about if the intervention is to be transferred from one setting to another. In other words, in health promotion where the issues involved are often highly complex and the settings difficult to control (unlike, say, a drug intervention conducted in a hospital setting), key information will often not be available from trial data. It also means that because of the way questions are set in RCTs, certain types of question, especially those relating to process or to potential mediating factors (which are deliberately controlled out of the RCT), remain unanswered or undescribed. Great care also has to be taken too when interpreting the literature, so that errors are not compounded.

The sixth and final issue is that when conducting reviews you also have to think about the problems of synthesizing evidence from different research traditions (Dixon-Woods *et al.*, 2004). As with all evidence work, the critical appraisal process used in compiling the evidence base has to focus on the question of thresholds of quality, or of grading the evidence. Not all evidence is of uniformly good quality, so the ways of discriminating between different qualities in evidence has been a preoccupation in much of the process itself. This applies equally to the quality of systematic reviews as to the quality of primary research studies (Swann *et al.*, 2003).

Getting research evidence into practice

Getting the evidence into practice is an even greater challenge because, as noted above, even the best quality scientific evidence does not say very much about factors that are significant in terms of making interventions work. Most reported studies say very little about how to do the intervention, at least in terms of what took place interpersonally, organizationally or politically. Process data about the ins and outs of the mechanics and problems associated with doing the intervention are also limited. The way that local infrastructures and local professionals engage with the process is underreported. What the intervention consisted of is frequently not included in reports. In fact, because of the imperative in modern science towards generalizability, specific local factors are precisely those which are controlled out of experimental designs. Consequently, the very information which sheds light on the mediating factors that determine the extent of success needs to be ascertained by some other method.

Local infrastructure such as the degree of involvement of professional groups, local organizational arrangements and local politics and leadership, all play critical roles in the success or otherwise of an intervention. This has led to a distinction between knowledge to be derived directly from scientific studies (which provide a framework of plausible accounts of why things work) and knowledge derived from practice (which helps understand the likelihood of success of an intervention). While there are tools to enable scientific studies to be graded according to their internal validity, it does not follow that valid evidence produces strong recommendations for action. Guidance and recommendations can only be made after an assessment has been made of the mediating factors operating on the ground and embedded in local practice. This assessment of the mediating factors is the type of knowledge which is concerned with the likelihood of success. A method to derive this information involves the collection of qualitative data from practitioners and attempts to understand local conditions (Kelly *et al.*, 2004a,b). So the evidence is seen as a framework of plausible possibilities and as a starting point for interventions rather than a recipe or imperative for action.

What the evidence suggests: two case studies

To illustrate reviews and synthesis of the evidence in health promotion, you will now read about two examples from the UK: accidental injuries and obesity. Each is subdivided into implications arising for implementation at national and at local level, segmented by setting where applicable. As well as being a summary of effective practice, they serve to illustrate some of the key lessons about evidence-based health promotion.

Accidental Injury (including fires)

These recommendations are based on three reviews conducted in the UK for the government agency responsible at the time, the Health Development Agency (Easterbrook *et al.*, 2001; Millward *et al.*, 2003; Mulvihill *et al.*, 2005).

Action needed at national level:

- Child-resistant packaging should be made compulsory on all actual or potentially poisonous substances.
- Smoke detectors that are hard-wired (rather than dependent on a battery) should be made compulsory in all new domestic dwellings and this provision should be incorporated into relevant building legislation.
- Selective breath testing and random breath testing sobriety checkpoints are both effective in preventing alcohol-impaired driving, alcohol-related crashes, and associated fatal and non-fatal injuries. The development of such policies should be regarded as a high priority.
- Laws enforcing a blood alcohol concentration (BAC) of 0.08 g/dl are effective in reducing alcohol-related crash fatalities. Lower concentrations are also effective in reducing alcohol-related crash fatalities among young or inexperienced drivers. The development of policies to reflect this should be regarded as a high priority.

Action needed at a regional level:

- Speed restrictions in urban residential areas should be actively pursued, paying special attention to issues of health inequalities in child pedestrian accidents.
- Comprehensive engineering schemes relating to kerbs, crossings and tactile and auditory signals should become the norm.
- There should be comprehensive police enforcement of speed restrictions on all roads.
- A legal duty should be imposed on local authorities, housing corporations and

private landlords to install hard-wired smoke detectors in all properties for which they are responsible.

Local:

- Trained staff should routinely deliver exercise programmes to all persons over the age of 70 living in their own home or in a residential home through the primary health care system. Home, pharmacological, medical and occupational therapy assessment must be made compulsory for all patients over 65 who have been treated in A&E departments for falls.
- Comprehensive pharmacological osteoporosis prevention programmes should be introduced in primary care.

School:

- Primary and secondary schools should implement integrated road safety education programmes.

Obesity

The following recommendations were based on a review conducted by Mulvihill and Quigley (2003).

National:

- The possibility of strict regulation or a total ban on the advertising and promotion of foods directly to children (including school–manufacturer link-ups for the purchase of school equipment and learning resources) should be urgently considered.
- Tax incentives to employers to encourage exercise and physical activity at and while getting to the workplace should be introduced.
- There should be a statutory requirement for local authorities and planners to create a healthy environment by carrying out health impact assessments of planning proposals. The environment will promote activity, provide access to healthy food choices and limit availability to less healthy choices/outlets for all people – particularly disadvantaged and vulnerable groups.
- A comprehensive and long-term nutrition strategy should be developed. This would require short-, medium- and long-term goals, supported by sufficient resources to deliver at the local level and to provide the necessary research. This would include a national strategy on obesity.

Local:

- The use of brief interventions in primary care for obesity management and healthy nutrition should be a routine part of all medical consultations.
- Specialist obesity treatment services for children and/or adults to which GPs can direct patients should be universally available. These services must provide services that deliver to disadvantaged and vulnerable groups in the population.
- Family-based behaviour modification programmes, where the whole family is involved where appropriate, incorporating diet, child management, parenting and communication skills, and activity and behaviour modification, should be provided.

- Adult-only based services that include diet, physical activity and behaviour modification should be made widely available.

Schools:

- Multifaceted school-based interventions which are integrated within a curriculum involving nutrition, physical activity, cooking, modification of school meals and tuck shops, teacher training, reduction in sedentary behaviour and behaviour therapy. This should include the prohibition of all snack products except water, fruit, milk and juice in school premises.

 Activity 15.2

These recommendations identify interventions that are known to be effective. Make a list of health promotion interventions that are used in your country but that do not appear on these lists.

 Feedback

You probably identified some additional health promotion activities in the fields of accidental injuries and obesity in your country. What these differences illustrate is the importance of local contextual factors in deciding on what measures are appropriate and feasible at any given time and in any given place. In other words, the scientific evidence as to what is effective is only part of the story. Just because some thing works in one place does not mean it will be successful elsewhere. In this way, evidence-based health promotion differs from determining what is the best drug treatment of a person with a particular disease.

 Activity 15.3

Using your list from Activity 15.2, what are the characteristics of the evidence-based and non-evidence-based interventions? Do you have any sense of which sort of interventions are the most successful? Are there any other characteristics about the interventions in each list? Does the list reflect the fact that it is easier to collect evidence about some things rather than others?

 Feedback

You will probably have generated a lot of examples of practice that are 'not' evidence-based, and yet you may know that on the ground they seem to be very successful. It is important to recognize that while it is essential to implement effective interventions where these are known and fit the circumstances, 'no evidence of effectiveness' does not necessarily mean 'not effective'. It may simply be that research has not been done in that area, or that the interventions are not amenable to experimental study. You will probably see that on your lists of 'no evidence' you have more upstream interventions rather than downstream-ones; more community-based rather than individual; more organizational or system changes rather than behavioural approaches for example. You should also have noted that the characteristics of the evidence in the areas of housing and working with communities differs from the more individual behavioural interventions featured in the health topic areas.

Summary

The call to develop an evidence base in health promotion has given rise to an important resource; for the first time, the evidence has been systematically mapped. There is still much to be done and new methodological and theoretical problems to be tackled. Two key issues figure highly: the problem of grading evidence in health promotion where the nature of the evidence is not strong and grading the recommendations derived from the evidence.

References

Cochrane AL (1972) *Effectiveness and Efficiency: Random Reflections on Health Services*. London: British Medical Journal/Nuffield Provincial Hospitals Trust

Dixon-Woods M, Agarwal S, Young B, Jones D, Sutton A (2004) *Integrative Approaches to Qualitative and Quantitative Evidence*. London: Health Development Agency (available at: http://www.publichealth.nice.org.uk/documents/integrative_approaches.pdf)

Easterbrook L, Horton K, Arber S, Davidson K (2001) *International Review of Falls in Older People*. A Report for the Health Development Agency. Centre for Research on Ageing and Gender, CRAG, University of Surrey

Graham H, Kelly MP (2004) *Health Inequalities: Concepts, Frameworks and Policy*. London: Health Development Agency

Hillsdon M, Foster C, Naidoo B, Crombie H (2004) *The Effectiveness of Public Health Interventions for Increasing Physical Activity Among Adults: A Review of Reviews*. London: Health Development Agency (available at: http://www.publichealth.nice.org.uk/documents/physicalactivity_evidence_briefing.pdf)

Kelly MP, Chambers J, Huntley J, Millward L (2004a) *Method 1 for the Production of Effective Action Briefings and Related Materials*. London: Health Development Agency

Kelly MP, Speller V, Meyrick J (2004b) *Getting Evidence into Practice in Public Health*. London: Health Development Agency (available at: http://www.publichealth.nice.org.uk/documents/getting_eip_pubhealth.pdf)

Millward LM, Morgan A, Kelly MP (2003) *Prevention and Reduction of Accidental Injury in Children and Older People: Evidence Briefing*. London: Health Development Agency (available at: http://www.publichealth.nice.org.uk/documents/prev_accidental_injury.pdf)

Mulvihill C, Quigley R (2003) *The Management of Obesity and Overweight: An Analysis of Reviews of Diet, Physical Activity and Behavioural Approaches. Evidence Briefing*. London: Health Development Agency

Wanless D (2004) *Securing Good Health for the Whole Population: Final Report, February 2004*. London: Department of Health

Glossary

Aim An expanded and refined version of a goal that sets out the means by which the end point, in general terms, is to be attained.

Aleatory uncertainty A situation in which you have fairly good knowledge of the probability of a particular outcome as it is known to be random.

Attribution Being able to relate a particular outcome to a particular cause.

Behaviour Actions, activities or conduct of people.

Beneficence Doing good; active kindness.

Community A neighbourhood and/or group with common interests and identity

Community A society, the population of a specific area, or groups of people. Can also refer to a neighbourhood, district or any centre of population.

Community development The process of change in neighbourhoods and communities. It aims to increase the extent and effectiveness of community action, community activity and agencies' relationships with communities.

Community participation A process by which individuals or groups assume responsibility for health matters of their community.

Context The circumstances surrounding an intervention, including cultural environment, political environment, existing work related to the intervention, current events shaping opinion on the topic, etc.

Effectiveness The extent to which an intervention produces a beneficial result under usual conditions.

Empowerment A central tenet of health promotion, whereby individuals are given knowledge, skills and opportunity to develop a sense of control and mastery over life circumstances.

Epistemic uncertainty A situation in which you have no knowledge of the probability of a particular outcome.

Evaluation The process of judging the worth or value of something.

Evidence-based medicine Movement in the medicine and related professions to base clinical practice on the most rigorous scientific basis, principally informed by the results of randomized controlled trials of the effectiveness of interventions.

Evidence-based practice The use of research evidence to guide practice, often associated with, but not synonymous with, the development of guidelines.

Evidence into practice The attempt to implement evidence in practice.

Final outcome evaluation Evaluation concerned with assessing the final outcome of a particular intervention in terms of its effect on the health of the target population.

Goal A general statement of intent, usually based on a set of principles or values.

Health The state of complete physical, mental and social well-being and not merely the absence of disease or infirmity.

Health belief model One of the first models of health behaviour change which focuses on the individual's calculation of risks and benefits.

Health promotion The process of enabling people to increase control over the determinants of health and thereby improve their health.

Healthy public policy An approach characterized by an explicit concern for health and equity in all areas of policy and an accountability for health impact.

Heuristics Problem solving by application of a method that generally yields reasonable solutions, as opposed to finding the best one.

Indicator An attribute or variable used in the measurement of change.

Inequalities in health Differences in health status between different population sub-groups.

Inter-sectoral collaboration Collaboration between organizations from different sectors working together to come to joint solutions about problems.

Intermediate outcome evaluation Evaluation that focuses on the behavioural impact (intermediate outcome) of an intervention.

Liberalism The rights of the individual should be respected to enable society on a whole to benefit from the full potential of all its citizens.

Message mapping Achieving message clarity and conciseness based on developing a consensus message platform, providing visual aids and road maps for displaying structurally organized responses to anticipated high concern issues, focused at specific stakeholder groups.

Model Simplified versions of something complex used to analyse and solve problems or make predictions.

Models of behaviour change Representations of how people think and act and the ways in which this can be changed; used to help predict and explain behaviour.

Motivation Incentives or driving forces that encourage the adoption of health-promoting behaviours or lifestyles.

Non-maleficence A principle based on avoiding the causation of harm.

Objective Concrete and specific elaboration of an aim.

Organizational capacity The human resources and management systems that an organization has.

Organizational climate The personality of an organization; those characteristics that distinguish one organization from another, based on the collective perceptions of those who live and work in it.

Organizational culture A set of values and assumptions about an organization.

Partnership Brings previously separate organizations into a more durable and pervasive relationship, with full commitment to a common mission.

Plato's republic Governance by those best qualified to do so.

Primary care Formal care that is the first point of contact for people. It is usually general rather than specialised and provided in the community

Process evaluation Evaluation that concentrates on examining the process of an intervention.

Programme development The design of an intervention with consideration given to identified needs, aims, objectives and contextual factors, such as cultural and political environment.

Programme evaluation Assessment of the value of a programme.

Programme implementation The act of applying a programme taking into account resources and target population.

Public health The science and art of promoting health, preventing disease and prolonging life through the organized effects of society.

Risk The probability that an event will occur within a specified time.

Salutogenic Health-producing or -promoting activities.

Social capital Facets such as sociability, social networks, trust, reciprocity and community and civic engagement.

Social classes Categories based on the occupation of the head of a household.

Social environment The settings, surroundings or atmosphere in which social groups or individuals live, work and interact.

Social inequities Differences in opportunity for different population sub-groups.

Social structures Ways in which society is organized, configured and constituted.

Socio-economic determinants Social and economic factors that influence health.

Standard The basis for comparison or a reference point against which other things can be evaluated.

Sustainability The extent to which an intervention may be continued beyond its initial implementation; this may be dependent upon a continued source of funding, programme effectiveness, or changing priorities.

Target Similar to an objective in that it usually contains a quantifiable measure set to be achieved by a particular date.

Target group The group to which an intervention is addressed.

Theory A set of interrelated propositions or arguments that help to clarify complicated problems or help to understand complex reality more easily.

Utilitarianism A theory of the good (whatever yields the greatest utility or value) and a theory of the right (the right act is that which yields the greatest net utility).

Index